eHEALTH AND REMOTE MONITORING

Edited by **Amir Hajjam El Hassani**

eHealth and Remote Monitoring
http://dx.doi.org/10.5772/3158
Edited by Amir Hajjam El Hassani

Contributors

Masako Miyazaki, Eugene Igras, Lili Liu, Toshio Ohyanagi, Pouyan Esmaeilzadeh, Lina F. Soualmia, Badisse Dahamna, Stéfan J. Darmoni, Duncan Sanderson, Marie-Pierre Gagnon, Julie Duplantie, Amine Ahmed Benyahia, Amir Hajjam, Vincent Hilaire, Mohamed Hajjam, Emmanuel Andrès, Ali Moukadem, Alain Dieterlen, Christian Brandt

Published by InTech

Janeza Trdine 9, 51000 Rijeka, Croatia

Copyright © 2012 InTech

Notice

Publishing Process Manager Vana Persen
Technical Editor InTech Prepress, Novi Sad
Cover InTech Design team

Additional hard copies can be obtained from orders@intechopen.com

eHealth and Remote Monitoring, Edited by Amir Hajjam El Hassani
p. cm.
ISBN 978-953-51-0734-7

For EU product safety concerns:
IN TECH d.o.o., Prolaz Marije Krucifikse Kozulić 3, 51000 Rijeka, Croatia,
info@intechopen.com or visit our website at intechopen.com.

Meet the editor

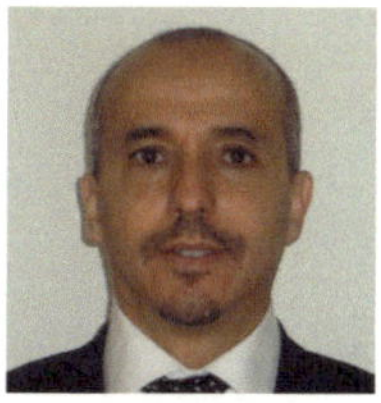

Dr Amir Hajjam El Hassani received his PhD in Computer Science from the Université de Haute Alsace in 1990. He joined the Université de Technologie de Belfort-Montbéliard in 2002. He performs research activities at the IRTES-SeT laboratory and is responsible for the research area of eHealth. He is Editorial Board Member of four international journals. He is the author/co-author of 3 books and many international publications in refereed journals and conferences. He was Co-Chair of the first international conference eTelemed'09 and is its advisory Chair since 2010. He is member of the Science Steering Committee of the annual conferences IADIS e-Health, eHealth, e-Medisys, etc. He has organised many conferences and chaired several technical sessions. He also acts as an expert to the ANRT France, ARI Alsace and CNRST Morocco.

Contents

Preface

In 1999, eHealth surfaced as a popular term referring to Internet-based health care delivery. Today, eHealth is making health care more efficient, allowing patients and professionals to do the previously impossible through the efficient Information and Communication Technologies (ICT). ICT are now used everywhere and play an important role in the delivery of high-quality and highly efficient health care services. Some eHealth applications have improved the quality of health care, and they are expected to lead to substantial cost savings in the near future. In today's digital society, ICT play an essential role in supporting daily life. eHealth initiatives, many of which are being undertaken in countries around the globe, have myriad benefits, including improvement of coordination and integration of health care delivery, empowerment of individuals and families for helping them manage their own health better and prepare health care plans, and facilitation of public health initiatives.

The ICT revolution has given rise to challenges with regard to health systems. The aim of this book is to present its impact on access to health care, quality of information on health care, cost-effectiveness of health care services and the development of eHealth equipment.

In chapter 1, we start with the challenges, strategies, and trends in eHealth. The authors discuss the opportunities and benefits associated with the adoption of eHealth solutions, as well as the impact of eHealth solutions on the health system and the population. eHealth services involving advanced technologies could have a significant impact on patient care in the future, including Internet-enabled applications for chronic disease management in the community. They could also facilitate self-monitoring of one's own health status. The authors show that eHealth will continue to evolve with advances in ICT, information science, medicine, and biotechnology. These topics are discussed in the Canadian context, but the discussions may be valid for other countries too.

A clinical decision support (CDS) system is an application that analyzes data to help health care providers make clinical decisions. In chapter 2, the author discusses the interactivity between physicians and CDS as the main variable affecting health care professionals who use CDS in their day-to-day activities. It shows that if health care professionals have an interactive relationship with a CDS, their level of involvement in the process increases and they have more control over procedures.

Most health care seekers, such as patients and their families (and even health professionals), are not familiar with the medical vocabulary, which is difficult to handle. Chapter 3 presents the main techniques used for improving information retrieval through health gateways.

The combination of EHR data and data generated through remote monitoring provides an important opportunity for following up the health of a patient. The increase in our ageing population is giving rise to new challenges in terms of disabilities and chronic diseases, incidences of which are expected to increase steadily in the coming years. Chronic diseases are ongoing, and generally incurable, illnesses or conditions, such as heart disease, asthma, and diabetes. They are the leading cause of death and disability in most developed countries. Admitting all these patients to institutions such as hospitals and nursing homes appears to be unfeasible. The general tendency is to provide homecare solutions involving remote monitoring, which offer unquestionably higher quality of care and greater security than conventional practices, and ultimately better quality of life for patients. In chapter 4, the authors present an architecture that combines the semantic Web and artificial intelligence, for homecare solutions. This architecture is based on generic ontologies so as to accommodate different conditions and types of sensors and data. A decision support base on an inference engine is used for following up the health of a patient and the detection of anomalies and abnormal situations and for responding appropriately, by providing recommendations and/or informing the patient's physician.

In the context of remote monitoring, the feasibility and accuracy of an Internet-based system for teleauscultation, involving the use of an electronic stethoscope, were evaluated. The results indicated that teleauscultation may be considered a reliable method for assessing cardiac patients. Chapter 5 reviews recent technological advances and presents an evaluation of promising innovations and perspectives in the field of auscultation. It focuses on the development of new intelligent communicating stethoscope systems in clinical practice and in the context of teaching and telemedicine. It shows that conventional auscultation is subjective and not easily shared. Modern medical technology allows us to optimize auscultatory findings and hence make a correct diagnosis by physically characterizing sounds through recordings, visualization, and automated analysis systems.

In a cardiac auscultatory system, many signals can be treated and monitored, e.g., ElectroCardioGram (ECG), PhonoCardioGram (PCG), Echo/Doppler and pressure monitor. The main point of interest in chapter 6 is the PCG signal. The author proposes a robust and generic PCG segmentation method that is useful in real-life conditions (clinical use, home care, professional use, etc.).

To date, some eHealth applications have improved the quality of health care, and they are expected to lead to substantial cost savings in the near future. However, eHealth is not simply a technology but a complex technological and relational process. In this sense, clinicians and health care providers who seek to successfully exploit eHealth should pay special attention to technology, ergonomics, human factors, and organizational changes associated with the structure of the relevant health service. We hope that this book will be useful to engineers, researchers, and industry personnel, and provide them with new ideas to address not only current issues that they are facing but also future issues.

Dr. Amir HAJJAM EL HASSANI
University of Technology of Belfort-Montbeliard,
Institute for Transportation Research, Energy and Society -
Systems and Transport, Belfort,
France

Chapter 1

Global Health Through EHealth/Telehealth

Masako Miyazaki, Eugene Igras, Lili Liu and Toshio Ohyanagi

Additional information is available at the end of the chapter

http://dx.doi.org/10.5772/47922

1. Introduction

EHealth is an umbrella term that covers Health Informatics, Telehealth and other ICT (information and communications technology) solutions in health care and medicine. It has been broadly defined as "the intersection of medical informatics, public health and business, referring to health services and information delivered or enhanced through the Internet and related technologies. In a broader sense, the term characterizes not only a technical development, but also a state-of-mind, a way of thinking, an attitude, and a commitment for networked, global thinking, to improve health care locally, regionally, and worldwide by using information and communication technology" [1].

EHealth also incorporates virtual reality, robotics, multi-media, digital imaging, computer assisted surgery, wearable monitoring systems, health portals.

While the primary focus of Health Informatics is the use of information systems and digital repositories in healthcare (electronic health record or EHR, medical terminologies, clinical guidelines), Telehealth refers to the use of ICT for the purpose of providing services across distance, time, social and cultural barriers. These services include both clinical services (such as telemedicine, telenursing, telerehabilitation, telepharmacy, teledentistry, or telemonitoring) and non-clinical applications (health education, research, or administrative). Telemedicine focuses primarily on the delivery of clinical care and includes a number of speciality terms such as teleradiology, telepathology, telepsychiatry, teledermatology and telesurgery. [2]

In this chapter we discuss the challenges, strategies and trends in healthcare. We also discuss the opportunities and benefits associated with the adoption of eHealth/Telehealth solutions as well as their impacts on the health system and the population. Although these topics are discussed in Canadian context, they may also apply in other countries.

One of the fundamental goals of health systems in most countries is to provide equitable access to healthcare. However, there are multiple and varying barriers to achieving this goal.

In some countries these barriers include limited access to portable clean water, a trained healthcare worker or critical lifesaving drugs. Other countries face challenges with providing medical intervention or an inoculation to prevent infectious diseases from spreading in an equitable and timely manner. There are also significant disparities between urban and rural healthcare. The barriers in the rural regions include "limited local expertise, resources, economic infrastructure, reimbursement for health services, as well as difficulties in retention and recruitment of health professionals, smaller population bases, isolation, and significant distances from needed expertise and service." [3].

With advancement of ICT and financial support, we may be able to reduce the disparities between regions regardless of availabilities of local resources. For example, Canada's First Nations people are not only affected by geographical isolation, but also by chronic poverty, under- or unemployment, substance abuse, limited opportunities for education and social advancement. Most reserves are located outside of major cities where all the social amenities are available, including sophisticated health care services. Over the past two decades the federal government has initiated a process of "transferring of control" to native communities and regional organizations. As a part, health care has become an integral aspect of aboriginal self-determination. In general, chronic care patients such as diabetics fare better at their home environment [4]

While we implement eHealth/ Telehealth services, we have to be cognisant of the needs for business continuity and disaster recovery plans and solutions. The current set up for eHealth/ Telehealth services is quite fragile as the disaster recovery plans do not exist or their implementation is not adequate.

Consequently, the scope of eHealth has been expanded. The World Health Organization (WHO) defines eHealth/ Telehealth/e-commerce as follows: "Tele-health includes surveillance health promotion and public health functions. It is broader in definition than tele-medicine as it includes computer-assisted telecommunications to support management, surveillance, literature and access to medical knowledge. Tele-medicine is the use of telecommunications to diagnose and treat disease and ill-health. Telematics for health is a WHO composite term for both tele-medicine and tele-health, or any health-related activities carried out over distance by means of ICT [5].

2. Definition of eHealth/Telehealth through scoping studies

The primary focus of eHealth/Telehealth is not technology. Rather, it is the adoption of the discoveries in medical sciences and advances in ICT to improve access to health services, and expand the range of these services from care to disease prevention to health maintenance to health education. The technology is just an enabler.

EHealth systems and services combined with organizational changes and the development of new skills create new opportunities to improve the healthcare system locally, nationally and globally through the collaboration and contribution of many stakeholders, including patients, health professionals, institutions, governments, researchers, academia and industry.

The healthcare system faces increasing pressure to improve health service delivery, health outcomes, and to contain healthcare costs regardless of economic status of the country. These challenges are directly linked to the changes in population demographic (e.g., ageing population, increased prevalence of chronic diseases), and increased expectations and needs for more equitable access to care, improved quality of care, improved health outcomes, and improved safety of care. Recently, these challenges have become more acute because of the shortages of healthcare professionals, complexity and accelerated communicability of diseases in many countries.

To address these challenges and meet the healthcare needs of population, many countries implement strategies that include establishing national health programs, improving health service delivery systems, fostering health maintenance and disease prevention, adopting proactive approach to management of healthcare resources, fostering research and innovation and adopting standardization and integration across the health systems.

Oh and colleagues [6] reported the results of scoping study by using the search query string "eHealth" OR "e-Health" OR "electronic health". They used the Medline and Premedline (1966-June 2004); EMBASE (1980-May 2004); International Pharmaceutical Abstracts (1970-May 2004); Web of Science (all years), Information Sciences Abstracts (1966-May 2004); Library Information Sciences Abstracts (1969-May 2004); and Wilson Business Abstracts (1982-March 2004); dictionaries and an Internet search engine. They concluded that the term eHealth encompasses a set of disparate concepts, including health, technology, and commerce. In the definitions of eHealth, technology was viewed both as a tool to enable a process, function, service and as the embodiment of eHealth itself (e.g., a health website on the Internet). They discovered that technology was portrayed as a means to expand, to assist, or to enhance human activities, rather than as a substitute for them [6].

Paré and his colleagues [7] had reviewed more than 65 telemonitoring studies in the United States and Europe. The study, entitled "Systematic Review of Home Telemonitoring for Chronic Diseases", concluded that home telemonitoring produces accurate and reliable data empowers patients and influences their attitudes and behaviours, and may improve their medical conditions. They concluded that home telemonitoring produces accurate and reliable data, empowers patients and influences their attitudes and behaviours, and may improve their medical conditions.

According to their study, the key clinical impact of implementing telemonitoring was a decrease in emergency room visits, hospital admissions, and average length of hospital stays. The effects of telemonitoring tended to be more consistent in pulmonary and cardiac studies than in studies on diabetes and hypertension.

3. Role of local, provincial, national governments and international organization in promoting e-health/ Telehealth

In order to implement comprehensive and over reaching e-health/ Telehealth service, it is vital to have all levels of governments and international organizations' cooperation and support. Governments as policy-making organizations, play a key role in formulating regulations, governing, financing, and regulating the health and business sectors.

EHealth was discussed at the United Nations World Summit on the Information Society in December 2003 and at the World Health Assembly in May 2005. The World Health Organisation (WHO) has established various eHealth initiatives, such as the WHO Global Observatory for eHealth (GOe) in 2005, which aims "to provide Member States with strategic information and guidance on effective practices, policies and standards in eHealth". The World Summit on the Information Society (WSIS), held with the participation of 175 countries (second phase, 16-18 November 2005, Tunis), affirmed its commitment to "improving access to the world's health knowledge and telemedicine services, in particular in areas such as global cooperation in emergency response, access to and networking among health professionals to help improve quality of life and environmental conditions".

The second global survey on eHealth was conducted by the GOe in late 2009 and was designed to build on the knowledge base generated by the first survey in 2005. While the first survey was general and primarily asked questions about the national level, the 2009 survey was designed to be thematic with far more detailed questions used to explore areas particular to eHealth. The survey has provided the GOe with a rich source of data that is being used to create a series of eight publications, the Global Observatory for eHealth series. GOe has release three reports to date: Telemedicine - Opportunities and developments in Member States; Atlas of e-Health country profiles; and m-Health. They are the most updated collection of survey data on eHealth from around the world. Over 800 eHealth experts and 114 counties have contributed to the data collection process. The mobile-Health (mHealth) survey was focused to identify the diverse ways mobile devices are being used for health around the world and their effectiveness. It is also to highlight the most important obstacles to implementing mHealth solutions and to examine if mHealth can overcome the 'digital divide'. Their report was released in June 2011. For the purpose of their study, GOe defined mHealth as a component of eHealth and support medical and public health practice by using mobile phone by capitalizing on a mobile phone's core utility of voice and short messaging service (SMS) as well as more complex functionalities and applications including general packet radio service (GPRS), third and fourth generation mobile telecommunications (3G and 4G systems), global positioning system (GPS), and Bluetooth technology [5].

It is valuable to have global data on eHealth adaption stages. The following Canadian example illustrates how adaption of eHealth/Telehealth intertwines the governments, health care providers, patients, public sectors and industries.

3.1. Canadian example

Every Canadian citizen has access to publicly funded healthcare, however, the manner in which the healthcare system is structured, funded and governed varies from province to province. While each province sets its own policies, strategies and priorities, some of the challenges are common across the country.

Issues Associated with Healthcare Delivery

- Geography: Canada is a country of over 34.6 million people spread across almost 10 million square kilometres. While the majority is concentrated in a several urban areas, a significant proportion is scattered across the land in hundreds of geographically isolated communities, many in areas of extreme climatic conditions. These factors pose serious challenges to the provision of health services.
- Ageing population: Seniors constitute one of the fastest growing groups in Canadian society. By 2041, about 23% of the population will be over 65, up from 12% in 1995. This growing portion of the population will inevitably require the devotion of a larger proportion of expensive health resources.
- Shortage of health professionals: There is a general shortage of healthcare professionals. That threatens the supply of and extends wait lists for some healthcare services.
- Inequitable distribution of health professionals: Most health service providers live and work in large urban centres. This contributes to acute shortage of health professionals in many smaller communities and rural areas where the provision of equitable access to health services is increasingly challenging.
- Patient safety: Several studies conducted by the Canadian Patient Safety Institute revealed that a significant number of patients experienced adverse events. One of the studies [8] revealed that an estimated 7.5% of patients admitted to acute care hospitals in Canada in the fiscal year 2000 experienced 1 or more adverse events. Also, 36.9% of these patients were considered to have highly preventable adverse events. Most of the patients who experienced adverse events recovered without permanent disability; their adverse events contributed to longer stays in hospital or temporary disability. However, a small but significant proportion of patients died or experienced a permanent disability as a result of their adverse events.
- Increasing prevalence of public health threats: The number of incidents of chronic diseases is increasing. Furthermore, emerging threats to public health such as SARS and avian flu require a pan-Canadian health surveillance system to provide critical information to support a rapid and effective response. These factors contribute to a high utilization of the scarce healthcare resources.
- Limited integration: Silos of care fail to provide patients and providers with timely and seamless access to the information they require and cause delays and needless duplication of services.
- Fragmented funding: Funding of health services is a complicating factor and a matter currently of intense scrutiny and considerable controversy. The division of political, managerial and fiscal accountability across provincial and federal lines has created tensions particularly around the question of the current level, and most appropriate future level of funding.
- Budget constraints: New treatments and technologies cost more and put additional demands on the strained healthcare budgets.
- Language barriers: Canada is a culturally diverse country, which has created some health care challenges. From the last national census, of 30 million people, 18 million

speak English, 7 million French and 5 million a mother-tongue other than English or French (official languages). Not being able to speak either official language is an obstacle for newcomers when seeking or obtaining healthcare.

Recent Trends in Delivery of Healthcare Services

Notwithstanding the provincial variations, several major trends have emerged that have a direct impact on adoption of eHealth. These trends include:

- Consolidation of services: Entails consolidation of healthcare services delivery, either through hospital amalgamation or regionalization.
- Integration of services: Integration of vertical health service delivery across the continuum of care primarily through regionalization.
- Co-operation among service providers: Entails organizing workflows in such a way that they support the individual patient care process and facilitate co-operation among service providers.
- Partnering: Third-party provisioning of health services through various mechanisms including outsourcing, shared service organizations and partnering between several healthcare organizations.
- Alignment of federal and provincial strategies: Alignment of provincial eHealth agendas and strategies with the strong involvement of Canada Health Infoway - a federal organization created to foster and accelerate the development of pan-Canadian electronic health information systems.
- Investment in eHealth: Strong senior-level support for eHealth solutions within healthcare organizations, regional health authorities and provincial ministries of health.

National Health Strategies for Health Information

In 2001, Canada Health Infoway was launched to develop Health Information Strategy and deploy information management and information technology solutions across the country. Infoway is an independent, not-for-profit organization whose members are 14 federal, provincial and territorial Deputy Ministers of Health.

Canada Health Infoway invests in partnership with provincial and territorial governments and regional health authorities across Canada to implement and reuse compatible health information systems that support a safer, more efficient healthcare system.

Infoway and its public sector partners have hundreds of projects, either completed or underway, delivering electronic health record (EHR) and point-of-service solutions to Canadians – solutions that bring tangible value to patients, providers and the healthcare system.

To accomplish its mission, vision and goal, Canada Health Infoway invests in health information technology solutions in priority areas, including the Registries, Interoperable Electronic Health Records, Diagnostic Imaging Systems, Drug Information Systems, Laboratory Information Systems, Public Health Surveillance, Telehealth, Innovation and Adoption, and Info structure.

Canada's total healthcare expenditure was approximated at $121.4 billion in 2003/2004 fiscal year and $140 billion in 2005/2006 fiscal year. Although the Canadian health system is described as publicly funded, nearly 30% of funding comes from non-public sources, such as insurance companies and individuals.

As indicated in the 2003 Report on Canadian Hospital IT: Top Issues, Applications and Vendors, less than 2% of healthcare funding in hospitals is spent on information technology majority of which (over 80%) is spent on maintaining existing infrastructure and only 17% is devoted to development of new information technology solutions.

Public spending on eHealth is heavily influenced by Canada Health Infoway. Canada Health Infoway is an independent not-for-profit organization whose members are Canada's 14 federal, provincial and territorial Deputy Ministers of Health.

For more detailed information see [9]

EHealth-Related Considerations:

While the initiatives led by Infoway and its public sector partners are an integral part of the pan-Canadian strategy to improve the health system, there are numerous challenges involved in the implementation of these initiatives. Examples include:

- Privacy and security: Concerns about personal privacy and information confidentiality and the recent proclamation of Privacy and Confidentiality legislation across the provinces and territories is a considerable challenge to the development of inter-jurisdictional data sharing arrangements and to storage and manipulation of data holdings (especially patient records).
- Standardization and interoperability: There is a growing recognition that compliance with health informatics and technology standards is critical to achieving interoperability among eHealth solutions. However, given the number of health informatics and technology standards, their state of maturity and adoption, and lack of universal interoperability standards for eHealth, the challenge of building plug-and-play interoperable systems requires significant expertise and continuing effort.
- Integration with service delivery: the integration of technology with the service delivery system is a key critical success factor for a wide adoption of eHealth solutions.
- Technology suitability: Deployment of eHealth solutions that are suitable and well-aligned with the healthcare workflows is critical. Some challenges still remain to be addressed. For example, some of the technologies remain unproven in extremes of climate and in far-north locations. There are also limitations imposed by the fragility and newness of certain technologies and products in situations where ongoing technical maintenance and operational services are limited or do not exist.
- Technology acceptance: Public and professional acceptance of the new technology solutions and new ways of service delivery remains a significant risk factor and a challenge to be addressed.

- Safety: while there is growing recognition that eHealth solutions assist in ensuring patient and health professional safety, there is also recognition that the safety of eHealth products must be addressed in a similar way as for medical devices.
- Sustainability: There is a growing recognition that the deployment of eHealth solutions goes beyond technology and involves change management and further investment. Financial and human resources must be invested in the management and operations of the eHealth solutions to realize their full potential and be sustainable.
- Education and training: Education of sufficient numbers of information technology, information management and health informatics specialists to implement, operate, manage and continue the development and improvement of the technologies and the systems remains a challenge that needs to be addressed.

The healthcare market is changing and expanding at a rapid rate and the focus is on automation, increased efficiency and effectiveness of decision making, improved outcomes and patient care provider safety through the increasing use of information technology and eHealth applications.

The following table presents some examples of trends in care delivery and eHealth/Telehealth solutions.

Future Global Healthcare Strategies is quite clear from the Canadian example that there are many challenges associated with an adoption of eHealth/Telehealth at the national level. There have been many pilot projects and initiatives using varied equipment and strategies. Some of the initiatives have been sustained and others were abandoned. The key factors for abandonment are costs and benefits, complexity of technologies, low level of acceptance among healthcare service providers, and lack of technical assistance.

Over a decade, Wootton had held annual conference on "Success and Failure of Telehealth" He found that despite the large number of published articles on the concept of telemedicine in the developing world, there are remarkably few examples of successful implementations. Wootton and others [10] have published a book on "Telehealth in developing world" which summarized the experience of starting and sustaining Telehealth projects in the developing world. This book has assembled large contribution of Telehealth experience from developing countries.

According to the International Telecommunication Union, there are now close to 5 billion mobile phone subscriptions in the world. In 2010, there were 143 counties which offer third generation mobile telecommunications (3G) services and several counties are even moving toward fourth generation mobile telecommunications (4G). The Internet access is essential for eHealth and two billion people are Internet users of which 1.2 billion are in developing counties [11]. Given the volume of available mobile phones in the world, the prospect of using mobile phone or devices for healthcare seems promising.

Therefore, it is reasonable for the WHO to pay special attention to mHealth, following the extensive survey of eHealth activities among the member countries. Fourteen categories of mHealth services were surveyed: health call centres, emergency, toll-free telephone services,

Trends	Examples of eHealth Solutions	Purpose
Consumer Health Informatics		
Client empowerment	Health information portals eLearning systems Collaborative tools	Provide access for health information and education material Connect to others who have the same / similar health conditions Participate in support groups
Self-Care	Personal electronic health record Monitoring devices and bio-sensors Medical devices eLearning systems	Collect data about health status Monitor health conditions and lifestyle Perform diagnostic procedures Perform non-invasive treatment interventions
Personal health record	Electronic health record / smart card Document management Data integration systems Messaging systems Privacy and security solutions	Collect data about health status Provide a comprehensive and secure clinical view of client health information accessible to authorized persons (e.g., healthcare professionals) from any location at any time
Evidence-based medicine	Electronic health record Good health practices Health information portals	Provide access to evidence-based guidelines, studies, and health practices Promote good health practices
Professional Informatics		
Computer-aided decision tools	Computer-aided clinical discipline / disease-specific practice guidelines Care pathways	Provide access to medical information / knowledge anywhere and anytime
Clinical communications	Electronic clinical communications tools for booking, referrals, clinical documentation	Communicate electronically with clinical systems and other services providers Assist in sharing clinical expertise
Knowledge management	Collaborative tools Multimedia conferencing systems E-learning systems Data mining tools Data fusion tools Rule discovery tools Knowledge capture systems	Organize and disseminate the existing knowledge Create new knowledge taking into account tacit and explicit aspects of knowledge

Trends	Examples of eHealth Solutions	Purpose
Evidence-based medicine	Computer-assisted clinical practice guidelines Electronic health record Good health practices Health information portals Clinical support systems	Combine the new knowledge with the existing practices and clinical standards Provide tools for rigorous scientific evaluation of collected facts Develop and disseminate practice guidelines and health practices Provide access to medical journals and studies
Service Delivery		
Remote sensing and monitoring	Bio-sensors and wearable products Implantable devices Smart medical devices Telemonitoring	Monitor individuals with critical / chronic conditions Monitor individuals who work / live in extreme conditions
Remote service delivery	Telehealth systems Telemedicine applications Telelearning	Improve access to health and education services for people living in areas with limited access to these services Facilitate collaboration among the health stakeholders, including service providers and service recipients Provide a tool for continuing medical / health education
Personalized care	New diagnostic and treatment modalities Genomic and molecular medicine technologies, including sequencing, genotyping, gene expression profiling, and protein engineering Specialized tools to identify and stratify health risks and recommend preventative measures for individuals	Participate in the development of care plans and assessment of the appropriateness of care Facilitate collaboration among the health stakeholders, including service providers and service recipients Predict and prevent diseases
Population-based care	Population identification and screening tools Specialized tools to aid in decision-making	Facilitate population based health planning Predict the evolution of disease in populations

Trends	Examples of eHealth Solutions	Purpose
Medication management	ePharmacy systems Electronic health record Drug interaction systems Drug dispensing devices	Identify and stratify medical risks and recommend preventative measures for population Prescribe and monitor remotely clients' compliance with the care plan Coordinate response to extraordinary population-wide risks (e.g., pandemic, environment contamination)
Virtual health team	Collaborative tools Multimedia conferencing systems Teleconsultation applications eLearning systems Knowledge management systems	Facilitate collaboration among health stakeholders, including: Communities of practice / interest Service providers across different care areas, including acute, community, continuing care, mental health and other areas
Healthcare Business Management		
Proactive business management	Data mining tools Workflow management Forecasting tools Best management practices	Mine and analyze clinical, organizational and economic information across facilities and service areas to monitor and measure efficiency and effectiveness of the health service delivery system Perform forecasting and service delivery planning Develop and disseminate best management practices
Data Management and Protection		
Data and information quality	Search engine tools Data cleansing tools Data mining tools Data fusion and rule discovery tools Pattern-based tools Ontology tools	Ensure quality of data and information (e.g., accuracy, completeness, consistency, clarity, currency, relevancy, timeliness)
Integration	Virtual electronic health record Middleware Integration broker	Provide access to data Facilitate data exchange between heterogeneous systems

Trends	Examples of eHealth Solutions	Purpose
	Messaging system Enterprise application integration system	Integrate systems at different levels e.g., network, data, application level
Security	Security tools Persistent security	Protect systems and networks through providing security services e.g., authentication, authorization, auditing Protect data, information, knowledge in the environment where security services may not be available

Table 1. Examples of eHealth trends and solutions

managing emergencies and disasters, mobile telemedicine, appointment reminders, community mobilization and health promotion, treatment compliance, mobile patient records, information access, patient monitoring, health surveys and data collection, surveillance, raising health awareness, and decision support systems. According to mHealth document [12], mobile phones are used to call a call center, emergency calls, medical consultations but not for health promotion or decision support or surveillance in developing countries. In case of disaster, they will use mobile phone or toll free call. As they move forward with mHealth, it is a vital importance to establish a policy for protecting privacy and security of health data [13].

According to Paré et al. (2011), implementation of mobile device with customized homecare nursing software helped to structure and organizes the nursing activities in patients' homes. There were 137 homecare nurses and they were asked to complete a structured questionnaire and 101 had completed (74% response rate).The nurses reported significant level of satisfaction with the quality of clinical information collected. A total of 57 semi-structured interviews were conducted and most nurses considered the software to be user friendly. A questionnaire was mailed out to approximately 1240 patients and 223 patients responded. They reported that nurses who used mobile computing device during their home visits seemed to manage their health condition better and provided superior homecare services. The use of mobile computing had positive and significant effects on the quality of care provided by homecare nurses.

4. Disaster recovery plan

As we move forward with the ICT supported healthcare, we must ensure the security, integrity, business continuity and recovery of healthcare data and services after a disaster, either manmade or natural. Advancement of technology and adoption of ICT solutions have contributed to escalating amount of digital data in business and public sectors. It is quite common for health care to be affected by earth quakes, fire, floods and severe storms in resource rich counties.

EHealth/ Telehealth networks can be destroyed or disabled in few seconds by natural disasters like in Japan. Numerous natural disasters such as tsunami, hurricanes, earth quakes, ice storms, tornados, forest fires or floods can significantly affect people's ability to access basic necessities, such as food, shelter, and healthcare regardless of economic status of the country. In addition, there are numerous active wars and battle zones around the world where basic livelihood have been threatened.

Over the past decades there has been a substantial increase in the number of people affected by disasters and the subsequent socio-economic losses. In 2007, 414 disasters resulting from natural hazards were reported. They killed 16,847 people, affected more than 211 million others and caused over 74.9US$ billion in economic damages. Last year's number of reported disasters confirmed the global upward trend in natural hazard-related disasters, mainly driven by the increase in the number of hydro-meteorological disasters. In recent decades, the number of reported hydrological disasters has increased by 7.4% per year on average. (Annual Disaster Statistical Review: Numbers and Trends 2007, Center for Research on the Epidemiology of Disasters).

Therefore, disaster recovery should be an integral part of planning, development and adoption of ICT solutions in health. It is not a matter of if, but when disaster is going to happen. It is essential to have a policy and a disaster recovery plan for eHealth

An example of such as a policy has been developed by eHealth Ontario (2009) which states;

"Business continuity management processes must be implemented to identify and limit to acceptable levels the business risks and consequences associated with major failures or disasters, considering both the disruption of eHealth Ontario services and the capability and time to resume essential operations.

The potential consequences of disasters, security failures, and service disruptions must be analyzed to determine the criticality of services and supporting IT infrastructure components.

Integrated plans must be developed, implemented, and tested to ensure that all critical business services are maintained or can be restored on a prioritized basis, to an acceptable level and within the required time-scales, in the event of failure. Business continuity commitments for critical services must be incorporated into Service Level Agreements with clients. Disaster Recovery plans should be tested annually.

Contingency plans must provide for the following [13]:

- timely restoration of service disrupted by a failure within a system, process, or function
- emergency recovery of service at an alternate location in the event of a disaster or prolonged outage at the primary site
- limited recovery of critical services in the event of major loss of staff."

The mission of the Organisation for Economic Co-operation and Development (OECD) is to promote policies that will improve the economic and social well-being of people around the world. The OECD provides a forum in which governments can work together to share experiences and seek solutions to common problems such as healthcare.

As identified by the OECD, there is "an absence, in general, of independent, robust monitoring and evaluation of programmes and projects" [14]. In this context, there is a very real need to benchmark for the first time in a consistent and comparable manner eHealth deployment, take-up, and impact in hospitals across the EU27.

The OECD [15] has used a case study approach to explore the various handicaps, incentives, enabling of secure exchanges of information, and the use of benchmarking in relation to eHealth with an aim to determine which practices can improve the adoption and use of ICT. It undertook six case studies, three of which were in Europe (the Netherlands, Spain and Sweden). Internationally, it also explored the situation in Australia, Canada and the United States of America (USA). This study therefore plays a vital role in discovering the eHealth deployment, take-up, and impact in hospitals across the EU27.

According to eHealth Benchmarking III [16] was prepared based on the result of survey conducted by Deloitte, in association with Ipsos Belgium and with the support of Diane Whitehouse of The Castlegate Consultancy, on behalf of the Information Society and Media Directorate-General European Commission (EC).

They had surveyed 906 acute hospitals; targeted Chief Information Officers (CIOs) in all the hospitals and Medical Directors in 280 of the hospitals: CIOs were asked about the availability of eHealth infrastructure and applications in their hospitals; whereas Medical Directors were asked about priority areas for investment, impacts and perceived barriers to the further deployment of eHealth. The survey was carried out in 2010 in all 27 Member States of the European Union (EU) and in Croatia, Iceland, and Norway [16].

Their method of data collection and analysis were clearly stated and processes of cross validation were included within and between the questionnaires for the Medical directors and CIOs. Within this study, they have inquired about their disaster recovery plan doe the acute hospitals in EU.

Disaster recovery implies the ability to recover those mission-critical computer systems that are required to support the business's continuity – in this case, the business is the hospital. There were more than 80% of the hospitals have an enterprise archive strategy for long-term storage and disaster recovery.

Enterprise archive strategies relate to "a comprehensive information archiving strategy aligned with an organisation's goals and performance needs.

All the hospitals surveyed in eight European countries (Austria, Croatia, Cyprus, Denmark, Estonia, Iceland, Norway, and Sweden) have an enterprise archive strategy for long-term storage and disaster recovery. The similar trend exists in Belgium, Germany, Spain and the UK. However France and Italy are both below the EU+ average. Of the hospitals that have an enterprise archive strategy, for most of them it is driven by the hospital's own strategy. Only in a few hospitals is it driven by national or regional healthcare IT programmes. "IBM - Information Lifecycle Management Services - Enterprise Archive - North America." [17].

Many of the hospitals in EU are operationalizing the disaster recovery plan within the hospital except Denmark, Ireland and Sweden are the only three countries where the strategy is driven by either regional or national health care IT program more than by the hospital's own strategy.

Due to the nature of the service, it is essential to restore hospitals' critical clinical information. In EU, almost half the hospitals' critical clinical information system operations can be restored within 24 hours in the event that a disaster were to cause the complete loss of data at the hospital's primary data centre. However, 10% of hospitals say that this can only be done in less than one week. Shockingly, 1% says that it would take up to a month and, even worse, in another 1% of hospitals it would take more than a month.

Immediate recovery is possible in more than half of the hospitals in Luxembourg and Sweden. More than nine out of ten hospitals in Austria, Bulgaria, and Sweden would restore data immediately or within 24 hours. The response time is longer than 24 hours for more than half of the hospitals surveyed in Finland, Greece and Norway.

5. Conclusion

EHealth/Telehealth will continue to evolve with advances in ICT, information science, medicine and biotechnology. The new generation of healthcare providers and patients will be far more comfortable with new technologies, new applications and services, and innovative service delivery methods. There is also a growing recognition that eHealth provides an opportunity for healthcare providers to improve health systems and transform them from the 'Diagnose and Treat' to 'Predict and Prevent' models.

Author details

Masako Miyazaki* and Lili Liu
University of Alberta, Canada

Eugene Igras
IRIS Systems, Inc., Canada

Toshio Ohyanagi
Sapporo Medical University, Japan

6. References

[1] Eysenbach, G (2001). What is e-health? J. med. internet. res. 3 (1). Available: http://www.jmir.org/2001/2/e20/. Accessed 2012 April 29.

[2] e-Health; Open Clinical (2011). Available: http://www.openclinical.org/e-Health.html. Accessed 2012 April 29.

---

* Corresponing Author

[3] Alverson, DC, Shannon, S, Sullivan, E, Prill, A, Effertz, G, Helitzer, D, Beffort, S Preston, A (2004). Telehealth in the Trenches: Reporting Back from the Frontlines in Rural America". Telemed. j. e-Health 10: Sup 2, S95 – S109. Available: http://hsc.unm.edu/som/telehealth/docs/telemedjournalarticle.pdf. Accessed 2012 April 29.
[4] Health Canada, 2011: http://www.hc-sc.gc.ca/fniah-spnia/index-eng.php. Accessed 2012 April 29.
[5] Global Observatory for eHealth series (2011). Health Canada, 1-3. Available: http://www.who.int/goe/publications/ehealth_series_vol1/en/; http://www.who.int/goe/publications/ehealth_series_vol2/en/index.html; http://www.who.int/goe/publications/goe_mhealth_web.pdf). Accessed 2012 April 29.
[6] Oh, H, Rizo, C, Enkin, M, Jadad, A (2005). What is eHealth: a systematic review of published definitions. J. med. internet res. 7(1). Available: http://www.jmir.org/2005/1/e1/). Accessed April 30, 2012.
[7] Paré, G, Sicotte, C, Moreault, M-P, Poba-Nzaou, P, Nahas, G, Templier, M (2011). Mobile computing and the quality of home care nursing practice. J. telemed. telecare. 17:313 – 317.
[8] Baker, GR, Norton, PG, Flintoft, V, Blais, R, Brown, A, Cox, J, Etchells, E, Ghali, WA, Henert, P, Majumdar, SR, O'Beirne, M, Palacios-Derfingher, L, Reid, RJ, Sheps, S Tamblyn, R (2004). The Canadian Adverse Events Study: the incidents of adverse events among hospital patients in Canada. JAMC 25.
[9] Pan-Canadian Health Information Privacy and Confidentiality Framework 2005. Available: http://www.hc-sc.gc.ca/hcs-sss/pubs/ehealth-esante/index_e.html.
[10] Wootton R (2008). Telemedicine support for the developing world. J. telemed. telecare. 14: 109–14.
[11] The world in 2010: ICT facts and figures. Geneva, International Telecommunications Union, 2010. Available: http://www.itu.int/ITU-D/ict/material/FactsFigures2010.pdf. Accessed 2011 May 13.
[12] .WHO. Mobile health (mHealth). Available: http://www.who.int/goe/mobile_health/en/. Accessed 2012 April 30.
[13] eHealth Ontario (2009). Available: http://www.ehealthontario.on.ca/pdfs/Privacy/Information_Security_Policy.pdf. Accessed 2012 April 29.
[14] OECDHealth at a Glance Europe 2010 (2010). Available: http://ec.europa.eu/health/reports/docs/health_glance_en.pdf.
[15] OECD Health Data 2011 (2011) Available: http://www.oecd.org/document/30/0,3746,en_2649_37407_12968734_1_1_1_37407,00.html
[16] eHealth Benchmarking III; SMART 2009/0022 (2011). Final Report; Deloitte & Ipsos Belgium. Available: http://ec.europa.eu/information_society/eeurope/i2010/docs/benchmarking/ehealth_benchmarking_3_final_report.pdf. Accessed 2012 April 29.
[17] Data and information management services – enterprise archive. Available: http://www-935.ibm.com/services/us/index.wss/offering/its/a1030346. Accessed 2012 April 2012.

Chapter 2

Interaction with Clinical Decision Support Systems: The Challenge of Having a Steak with No Knife

Pouyan Esmaeilzadeh

Additional information is available at the end of the chapter

http://dx.doi.org/10.5772/48350

1. Introduction

Organizations invest in IT systems with the hope of cutting costs, increasing the quality of products or services [1]. But if users do not accept the systems, the organizations can not benefit significantly from the new systems. On the other hand, if users accept new IT systems they become more willing to make use of the new systems [2]. The usage of a newly introduced system can be a sign of the IT system success [3]. Therefore, finding the reasons that motivate people to use or understand the source of resistance to use new IT systems, is important to both system designers and developers [4].

The use of IT in health care practices has increased recently [5]. A variety of IT systems such as clinical information systems, personal digital assistants, electronic patient records and other applications have gradually become established in the healthcare industry. Clinical IT applications in healthcare are regarded as a key element in raising the quality of medical care. However, factors affecting the healthcare professionals' adoption behavior regarding IT systems are not completely clear yet [6,7,8]. The concern of having new clinical IT systems unused is still one of the biggest issues for the clinical IT developers [9,10].

With reference to a study done by Walter and Lopez [8] two types of IT are available in medical care environment. The first one is Electronic Medical Records (EMR) systems which are computer systems that allow users to create, store, and retrieve patient charts on a computer. The second one is Clinical Decision Support (CDS) system that is classified as a decision support system. A CDS System is regarded as an application of Decision Support System (DSS), which takes patient data as input and generates decision- specific advice [11,12]. These systems are referred to as knowledge-based systems that use patient data and series of reasoning techniques to generate diagnostic and treatment options and care planning. Typically, clinical IT is designed to enhance decision-making in health care environment and in this study the emphasis is on CDS systems.

There is enough evidence to state that healthcare professionals are different from other IT users in terms of accepting technology and may respond differently to clinical IT [13,14]. Their different IT adoption behavior is attributed to their professional characteristics such as specialized training, professional autonomy and professional work context. Healthcare professionals are highly sensitive to changes in their work setting especially they are more concerned about the kind of changes that are perceived as a threat to their professional autonomy [15,16,17,18]. On the other hand, different features of CDS such as guidelines and instructions given by those systems can affect healthcare professional's IT acceptance.

It means that the healthcare professionals' CDS adoption may be affected by their perceived level of interactivity with the CDS system. Therefore, the feature and nature of instructions and guidelines given by IT to healthcare professionals in terms of problem-solving process may be considered as an element that invalidate their professional autonomy [19]. Thus, the antecedent of healthcare professionals' perceived threat to professional autonomy is the rules, instructions and diagnostic options provided by the CDS.

2. Theory of professionals

While a variety of definitions for the term professional have been suggested, this study uses the definition from sociology. According to the classic work of Larson [19], professionals are defined as "members of occupations with special power and prestige based on special competence in esoteric bodies of knowledge linked to central needs and values of the social system". With attention to the study conducted by Sharma [20], members of some professions have been called professionals, in light of their command of focal as well as demanding knowledge that they possess. This list includes the holders of five professions namely financial analysts, lawyers, university professors, accountants and finally physicians.

It should be mentioned that generally, the medical profession has been thought of as the model or symbol of professionals based on the nature of the knowledge owned by physicians compared to the others. According to Watts [21] in all public polls which were taken in the USA in the second half of 20th century, the public selected physicians as the most honored professionals.

3. Types of healthcare professionals

In this study, the focus is on IT adoption behavior of healthcare professionals. Based on a review a literature, different types of medical workers are considered as healthcare professionals. Generally, healthcare professionals or medical professionals are distinguished from others as professionals specialized in serving diagnosis and treatment to patients' medical issues and disease. This group encompasses all physicians such as general practitioners, internists, pediatrics, radiologists, geriatrics, gynecologists, pathologists, surgeons, and other specialty doctors. For the entire mentioned group, the possibility of working with clinical information systems to deliver proper treatment and health care to patients is reasonable.

4. The unique characteristics of healthcare professionals

Professionals have some distinct and professional characteristics whereby they are viewed different from other non-professionals. Due to the scope of this study, the special characteristics of healthcare professionals are put at the center of attention. Healthcare professionals' professionalism has long been based on a defined set of values. The most important feature is healthcare professional autonomy and the other features are patient sovereignty, physician confidentiality, and habits of learning. According to Raelin [22], professional autonomy is defined as the control that professionals have over the processes and content of their work.

Patient sovereignty is defined as paternalism or the traditional model of doctor-patient relationship that includes official instruction and the patient's values in shared decision-making is not really emphasized in this type of communication [23]. Physician confidentiality is an important issue in the relationship between patients and physicians specifically in the disclosure of a patient's personal health information, medical histories and symptoms to physicians without any distress.

The increasing body of medical knowledge is a main concern to all types of doctors. Their habits of learning are associated with their subjective ability to keep themselves professionally updated on new medical findings. This includes spending time on attending courses/congresses and medical readings [24].

With reference to the findings of an exploratory study conducted by Chau and Hu [25], some unique characteristics are believed to be held by healthcare professionals. Three characteristics have been proposed as the main characteristics of this group. The first one is specialized training that reveals their domination over knowledge which has been obtained during a lengthy period of education. As stated by Watts [21], they devote a considerable portion of their youth preparing for the profession. Their body of knowledge is directly associated with the lives of patients. In this profession even a slight mistake can be fatal. Therefore, the heightened emphasis has been placed on specialized training of healthcare professionals.

The second characteristic is professional autonomy. Based on this characteristic, healthcare professionals proclaim that they are in the best position to drive, organize, and regulate their own practice. They are judged mainly through a peer review process in which professionals evaluate each other. As mentioned by Zuger [26], professional autonomy has clearly been the most important value. This advantage provides healthcare professionals with a sense of pride, and accomplishment. In addition, they take special power, prestige, and authorities, as well as they are put at the top of the hierarchy in the health care profession.

As stated by Watts [21], and Montague et al. [27], the last item is professional work arrangements where healthcare professionals become health care providers, hospitals became health care facilities, and a patient acts as both the product and the client in such a system. Also, in this setting, two other occupational groups (para-professionals and non-professionals) work with healthcare professionals. These two groups, the role they play in healthcare organizations and their relevance to this study is addressed in the following section.

5. Professional autonomy: The central privilege

According to Starr [28] at the start of the second half of the 20th century, healthcare professionals are viewed as the holders of desirable autonomy and respect within the health care industry. In accordance with Abbott [29], being members of a profession is certainly conducive to professional autonomy. Based on a study by Adams [30], professional autonomy is considered as a key factor of the medical profession. Drawing on a recent study by Walter and Lopez [8], professional autonomy is viewed as a precious privilege given to professionals and they do not like to lose it in their workplace. Throughout this research the term professional autonomy is used to refer to having control over the state of affairs, course of actions, practices, or components of their work in relation to their own collective and finally, individual conclusion for applying their profession's body of knowledge and capability [31].

As pointed out by Freidson [32], based on professional autonomy which is granted to professionals, individuals outside the profession (non-professionals) do not know how to evaluate the practices of the professionals due to lack of required knowledge. Relying on professional autonomy, physicians are provided with separate bylaws and arrangement within hospitals [28].

Professional autonomy generates two main expectations of professionals. On the one hand, they are required to practice with extreme conscientiousness and without any direct surveillance. One the other hand, they are trusted to take on the necessary measures in carrying out their tasks [33]. Previous studies have reported that it is very difficult to evaluate the physicians' performance due to the unstructured nature of their practice [34]. This view is supported by Wilson et al. [35] who point out that some usual objective measures like revenue or number of published articles, which are applicable to measure individual outputs in other practices, cannot be used to evaluate professionals especially physicians.

A peer review process is being utilized in professional settings in order to validate the evaluation of professionals based on subjective analysis of objective measures. According to Walter and Lopez [8], one of the most important characteristics of professional autonomy is being analyzed by peers instead of non-professionals who are outside the profession. Therefore, it is becoming increasingly difficult to ignore the importance of professional autonomy that indicates the possession of esoteric body of knowledge which the outsiders are not aware of.

On the basis of having professional autonomy, professionals are given some special rights. First, professionals take advantage of having more access to critical resources than non-professionals. A survey conducted by Freidson [33] shows that as long as professionals are not provided with adequate resources such as equipment and staff, they can claim that their work cannot be accomplished in the best way.

Second, professionals have power over the tasks carried out by non-professionals (ones who do not have professional qualification, skills as well as knowledge and are involved in administrative duties, clerical and office work) and para-professionals (ones who possesses only partial professional skills such as technicians that assist professionals in performing their work) and can control the tasks carried out by them [36].

It should be added that the advantage of having control over subordinate groups is more considerable in those organizations with existing hierarchies among various working groups. A hospital is regarded as an organization in which different work-related groups (physician assistants, nurses, medical technicians, and administration) possess different levels of medical knowledge and among all; physicians are placed at the top of the hierarchy. The following figure (Figure-1) shows the hierarchy of different occupational work groups involved in a hospital, based on their level of medical knowledge.

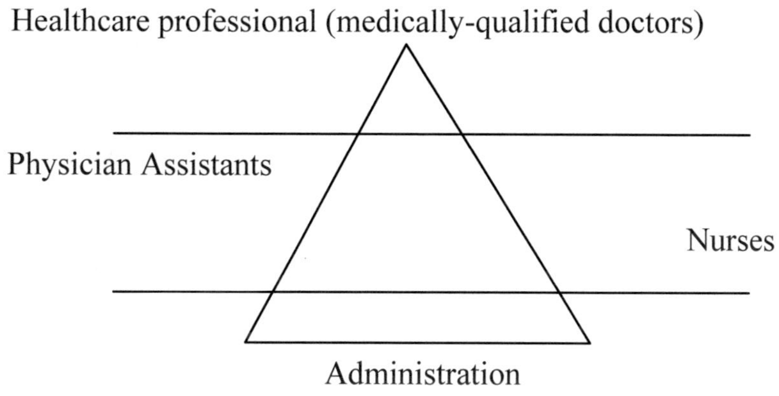

Figure 1. The hierarchy in healthcare organizations based on level of medical knowledge

6. Theory of interactivity

One view toward any new computerized system is that IT can reduce dependence on specific personnel [37]. These rules, procedures, and recommendations designed and embedded in IT can weaken their claim on possession of special competence in problem solving. Moreover, these instructions can invalidate their decision making skills in terms of deciding what to do for treatment of their patients. As stated by Harrison et al. [38], healthcare professionals feel uncomfortable when they face regulations and instructions generated by a clinical decision system that advises them on what to do. This is because they believe that they can treat their patients based on their specialized knowledge, experience, skills and competence. According to Lowenhaupt [39], healthcare professionals become more anxious when someone or something (such as a computer system, here is CDS) shows he/it has more knowledge than them regarding what to be done with their patients.

Bucy [40] has mentioned that there is a slight difference between interactivity and social interaction in the form of person-to-person conversation or face-to-face communication. On the one hand, interactivity can be viewed as a special sort of mediated social interaction, like online chat, discussion forums, or teleconferencing. On the other hand, it can appear as impersonal interactions with media content or nonhuman agents such as computer game playing, e-commerce transactions, and various other forms of content interactivity. Perceived level of interactivity is largely based on the belief that the interactive nature of the clinical system can assist in creating cooperation between healthcare professionals and clinical IT systems. Perceived level of interactivity with CDS can be divided into three parts. 1. Interactive features of CDS itself. 2. being responsive to customized needs of healthcare professionals. 3. Interaction between healthcare professionals and CDS.

In this study, the effect of level of healthcare professionals' interactivity with a new CDS is examined on the perceived threat to professional autonomy. Based on the interactivity theory which explains human – computer perceived interaction; a high level of interactivity can be demonstrated in simultaneous, reactive and continuous exchange of information [41] that assists in conducting users' tasks. A higher perceived level of interactivity with a system causes higher degree of control that healthcare professionals have during the interaction with an IT system. Higher level of control consequently may result in the less threat perceived from the system to their professional autonomy and in turn they become more prone to use the new IT. This issue indicates that when healthcare professionals perceive low level of control over the health care process due to the function and features of the new CDS, they become less likely to use the system. In other words, if healthcare professionals perceive that the regulations given out by CDS may threaten their professional autonomy and CDS acts as their supervisor directing them what to do without their interference, they perceive this kind of IT (with low level of interactivity) as encroaching on their professional autonomy. Thus, different level of interactivity with CDS system is conducive to different perception toward using that system. For instance, healthcare professionals may perceive a low level of interactivity with the CDS in comparison with the EMR.

As a result, perceived level of interactivity is largely based on the belief that the interactive nature of the clinical system can assist in creating cooperation between the healthcare professionals and the IT system. If healthcare professionals perceive that the nature of new CDS is interactive, they perceive more control and in turn they perceive less threat to their professional autonomy [8]. As a result, we propose that low level of perceived interactivity with CDS leads to low level of involvement in performing activities with the aid of the CDS system. Therefore, this situation inevitably results in low level of perceived control over processes and procedures of patients' treatment.

Interactivity has been defined in the literature in diverse ways [42]. Based on a review of the literature, interactivity is generally delineated as a property of the technology, the communication setting, or the perceptions of users [43]. In the first part of the definition, features of technology provide the set of interface actions that the systems allow and the degree of interaction changes based on user skills and competencies. The second part of the definition points to the communication setting as the locus of interactivity and specifies that interactive processes can be observed in the form of message exchanges (e.g., [44]). The control that users practice over the content of mediated exchanges is at the core of both message-related and technology-oriented definitions of interactivity.

According to Steuer [45] interactivity is defined as the "extent to which users can participate in modifying the form and content of a mediated environment in real time". Likewise, Neuman [46] stated that interactivity is "characterized by increased control over the communication process by both the sender and receiver". Williams, Rice, and Rogers [47] put forward interactivity as "the degree to which participants in a communication process have control over, and can exchange roles in, their mutual discourse". Based on Jensen [48] interactivity is "a measure of a media's potential ability to let the user exert an influence on the content and/or form of the mediated communication'. In the media literature, interactivity is regarded as a key motive for users' social responses to computers [49].

Stromer-Galley [50] has brought up the matter of categorizing the different types of interactivity into two general dimensions: interactivity as a product and interactivity as a process. The first type is related to interaction with content, dealing with the control that users apply over the selection and presentation of online content, such as text, audiovisuals, multimedia, and other features of the interface [50]. McMillan [43] has mentioned that product interactivity is a type of user-to-system interaction, whereas Stromer-Galley [50] previously used the term media interaction. Also Rafaeli [51] call such interactions as reactive communication. The second type of interactivity addresses person-to-person conversations which are mediated by the technology. Massey and Levy [52] have called this process interpersonal interactivity. McMillan [43] has employed the term user-to-user for this form of interaction while Stromer- Galley [50] referred this to the human interaction.

According to McMillan and Hwang [42], three elements come out commonly in the interactivity literature: direction of communication (responsiveness and exchange), user control (participation and features) and time (timely feedback and time required for retrieving information). Many studies have taken Human-to-Computer Interaction (HCI) into account to explain the ways humans can gain control over computers and other new media, such as video games [53, 54]. Reeves and Nass [49] have stated that with attention to user control, a group of scholars centers their studies on human perception and another group focuses on computer design. As far as a human focus is concerned, studies examine how individuals interpret computer character [55]. Interactivity acts to provide a human-like signal in the context of human-computer to fill the interface with agency and motivate users to communicate with the computer not only as a medium but also as a source of interaction [56].

Interactivity has some positive consequences in relation to user-system behavior. The level of interactivity might be vital to get users be involved in the online process, hence interactivity may make consumers more alert about information when working online [57]. Based on Bucy [58], the positive benefits of interactivity usually referred to as increased engagement, knowledge gain (or uncertainty reduction), user satisfaction, and efficacy. Other studies have stated that increased interactivity leads to increased feelings of tele-presence [59], greater involvement with the system [44], and creating more positive attitudes toward the system such as higher credibility [60]. As stated by Agarwal and Karahanna, [61] a greater sense of involvement with an IT system reduces the perceived cognitive burden and encourages the user to spend more time experiencing the system.

7. Healthcare professionals' perceived level of interactivity with clinical IT system

The interactivity construct has been initially focused on the context of computers, websites, online advertisements, and web-based mass communication but it has not been tested yet with technologies and IT applications in other fields especially in professional environment. In this study, the concept of interactivity is extended from the context of interaction between customers and websites as well as online advertising to clinical information systems and the healthcare professionals. Therefore, this study is a step forward in defining the concept of interactivity with clinical information systems and extending it to the professional context of healthcare practice. In the context of this study, interactivity can be defined as the amount and quality of two-way communication, reciprocal activity, cooperation and direct relationship between the CDS and healthcare professionals when the CDS asks requirement and disease symptoms to operate based on the built in instructions. One of the antecedents of physicians' perceived threat to professional autonomy is the rules, instructions and diagnostic options provided by the CDS. Function of any new computerized system (such as CDS) can reduce dependence on specific personnel [72]. But the culture of medical practice has always given emphasis to individual physician autonomy [73,74]. Therefore, maintaining the autonomy causes the changes brought by IT systems not to be always well-received by healthcare professionals and becomes one of the biggest challenges for CDS implementation in particular. Also, concerns about overreliance on the device (CDS), makes healthcare professionals become worried on losing their autonomy. According to Lowenhaupt [39], physicians become more anxious when someone or something (such as a computer system) can perform in a way as though he/it knows more than physicians do about their patients. As a result, they feel their level of control over patient care process, decisions and resource allocation will become less by the presence of the CDS. On the other hand, rules, procedures and recommendations designed and embedded in CDS can be seen as encroaching on the healthcare professionals' professional autonomy. As stated by Harrison et al. [38], physicians feel uncomfortable when they are faced with regulations and instructions produced by CDS advising them what to do because they believe they are able to treat their patients better based on their specialized knowledge, experience and competence. According to the study conducted by Dowswell [14], a majority of general practitioners accepted clinical guidelines as a tool to enhancing healthcare delivery, but when they perceived the encroaching guidelines on their professional autonomy, they started showing negative reaction toward the IT system.

On the one hand, Pain et al. [65] have stated that a computerized prescription system cannot eliminate the power of the doctor, because at the end of the day the doctor has the authority to decide what medicine to be prescribed. On the other hand, as suggested by Walter and Lopez [8], features of a clinical information system may influence perceived threat to professional autonomy. One possible feature is the level of interactivity that may change user perception of control and consequently affect perceived threat to professional autonomy. In the context of healthcare, perceived control can be described as the amount of control that a physician feels she/he has in using a clinical information system. Healthcare professionals' resistance toward using CDS does not always occur because the CDS distributes their abstract knowledge among the subordinate group in a hospital setting. Most of the time the rules and recommendations given by the system make healthcare professionals feel threatened because the system itself invalidates their exclusive knowledge claim. According to Mclaughlin and Webster [66], lab officers and medics perceived rules and recommendations of the IT system as threatening to their professional autonomy. Some respondents in this study declared that they changed the way the system interacted with them in order to save their autonomy.

Therefore, one feature of clinical information systems that influences professionals' perceived control is their level of interactivity. Perceived interaction is characterized as the level of interaction that a user perceives while experiencing the computerized system, and the extent to which the system is perceived to be responsive as well as sensitive to the user's needs. With attention to the medical literature, there are three levels of interactivity with a medical technology [67]. At the first level, healthcare professionals use the technology as a means to generate data so the experts can make a diagnostic decision. Therefore, at this level of interaction the medical IT can be considered as an enabler. At the second level, the technology is more complicated and acts as a partner of professionals. At this level both physicians and technology have the same weight. At the third level, the role of healthcare professionals is demonstrated in supervising the technology. At the third level, the technology takes on decision making process and recommends course of action and users are just responsible to control the process. At this level healthcare professionals are considered as operators. According to Lacramioara and Vasile [68], a factor that plays an important role in the interaction between human and computer for healthcare applications is the functionality of a simple, responsive and useful user interface. Also as stated by Tung et al. [6], information quality and message prompting have found to be influential factors.

Perceived level of interactivity with CDS can be divided into three parts. 1. Interactive features of CDS itself. 2. being responsive to customized needs of healthcare professionals. 3. Interaction between healthcare professionals and CDS.

1. The features of CDS's information delivery such as quality of information and basic evidence are the most important causes for the effect of CDS on patient safety and quality improvement. A question arises in this area is how much control the user will have in getting access to the CDS information. According to Osheroff [69], the "five rights" of CDS is a good guideline of what is required for having effective delivery. CDS should be designed in a way to give the right information to the right person in the right format through the right channel at the right time (when the information is needed).

The key issues for healthcare professionals to consult with a patient using the CDS are speed and ease of access. Users may be aware of the need for information but if access is too difficult or time-consuming, healthcare professionals may prefer not to use the CDS.

2. The interactive CDS includes both nationally recommended guidelines and customized order sets designed by an individual healthcare professional [69]. Therefore, the interactive CDS is responsive to the needs of healthcare professionals in unique case of a patient and encompasses order sets adapted for particular conditions or types of patients (ideally based on evidence-based guidelines and modified to manifest individual healthcare professionals' preferences).

According to Berner [70], the CDS that is integrated into the workflow and work activities is more likely to be used by healthcare professionals. On the other hand, fitting CDS features (such as timing, structure, and design) into the workflow often necessitates unique customization to local processes and configuring the system for use in the local environment. In some case where the previous clinical processes were inefficient or ineffective, the processes should be changed. According to Miller et al. [71], in some cases, some special features of CDS are ordered to fit into the local context.

3. Healthcare professionals should be involved in entering patient data into the CDS application and also getting relevant information (e.g., lists of possible diagnoses, drug interaction alerts, or preventive care reminders) from the CDS to perceive more control over the care processes. On the other hand, if the CDS's recommendations and notifications are delivered but the healthcare professional does not interact with the system, the effect of timely response is doomed to be a failure [71].

A question related to autonomy is how much control healthcare professionals have over the system and how they respond to the CDS. This aspect of control relates to whether it is mandatory for them to accept the CDS suggestions, whether they can easily not take the suggestions into account, or whether the healthcare professionals take significant effort to override the CDS advice [71]. Previous theories of CDS gave more emphasis to CDS output and limited healthcare professionals' control, but the new methodology of using CDS states that healthcare professionals can filter, review and finally select the useful and relevant suggestions and override others. With the use of this method a balance between healthcare professionals' desire for autonomy and the CDS suggestions for improving patient safety or decreasing practice costs, is made.

To sum up, the main goal of CDS is to interact with healthcare professionals and assist them in providing care planning and diagnosis analysis. In this human-machine interaction, both the healthcare professional's knowledge and the CDS function are required to better analyze the patients' data rather than relying on either human or CDS to make it on their own. In the interactive relationship between CDS and health care professionals, healthcare professionals input a set of required information and CDS makes a set of suggestions, advice and diagnostic options for the healthcare professionals and they go over the output and select useful one and remove irrelevant suggestions. In this manner, a CDS does not make decisions for healthcare professionals telling them what to do. Also, the process of interaction with CDS can be perceived more interactive when the possibility of adapting and customizing the system is considerable in case of a patient. Therefore, in this way healthcare professionals perceive CDS as an enabler or partner in which the decisions are not directly made by the CDS system.

Perceived level of interactivity is largely based on the belief that the interactive nature of the clinical system can assist in creating cooperation between healthcare professionals and clinical IT systems. According to McMillan and Hwang [72], by improving understanding on perceived interactivity, kind of systems can be developed that effectively make use of interactivity. If healthcare professionals perceive that the nature of new clinical system is more interactive, they perceive more control over process. As a result, the possibility of interaction with the system increases and in turn lowers their perceived threat to the professional autonomy. Psychologists argue that the feeling of being in control of any stimulating event results in approaching behavior, while a lack of that makes anxiety and leads to avoidance behavior [71]. According to Pianesi et al. [73], following the suggestion of Hoffman and Novak [74], it is shown that higher levels of involvement result in a greater feeling of being in control. As stated by Prasad and Prasad [75], employee involvement in interaction with systems can minimize resistance to technological change in organizations.

Thus, different level of interactivity with IT system is conducive to different perception toward using that system. For instance, healthcare professionals may perceive low level of interactivity with the CDS in comparison with the EMR because they think their role in the decision making and treatment gradually becomes less significant while using CDS.

8. Conclusion

As mentioned before, one way to reduce perceived threat to professional autonomy is directly related to organizational environment and human-human relationship such as the healthcare professionals' relationship with other occupational groups like the subordinate group. The second way to decrease the negative effect of perceived threat to professional autonomy is related to machine-human interaction and the structure, instructions and features of a CDS system [8]. As literature states, a new CDS can reduce dependence on healthcare professionals. Therefore, healthcare professionals are always worried about overreliance on CDS and consequently losing their autonomy. In this regard, the rules, recommendations, instructions and care planning provided by a CDS is another base for healthcare professionals to view CDS as threatening to their professional autonomy and make them believe they are losing their control over the processes, procedures of their practice.

To reduce this negative effect, the study recommends high level of interactivity with the CDS system. Interactivity is characterized by increased control over the relationship between user and system. Higher level of interactivity leads to a higher level of involvement with the system and increase the control over each step of the patient care process [44]. Also, the high level of interactivity encourages the users to spend more time experiencing with the system. In another view, interactive nature of a CDS system can assist healthcare professionals in creating a reciprocal relationship with the system. If healthcare professionals perceive that the nature of a CDS system is interactive, they perceive more control over the process.

This study is one of the first attempts to examine the construct of perceived level of interactivity as a means to reduce the negative effect of perceived threat to professional autonomy among healthcare professionals. The result of this study shows that if healthcare professionals have an interactive relationship with the CDS system, their level of involvement in the process increases and they believe more control over the procedures. Under this situation, instead of showing negative reaction toward new CDS they support the new system in hospital. As a conclusion, the more interactivity perceived by healthcare professionals, the less threat perceived from the new CDS system. This result has a practical implication for IT design. One way to reduce perceived threat to professional autonomy is directly related to user-machine relationship and features of the CDS system. One important aspect of interactivity is rooted in the features and instructions embedded in the CDS system. The interactive features of the system increase interactivity which is perceived by healthcare professionals in the relationship with the system. Based on the findings, IT designers should design the features, rules and instructions of the CDS system more interactive in order to increase the healthcare professionals' level of control over the patient care process.

Author details

Pouyan Esmaeilzadeh
Graduate School of Management, Universiti Putra Malaysia (UPM), UPM Serdang, Selangor, Malaysia

9. References

[1] Lederer, A.L., Maupin, D.J., Sena, M.P. and Zhuang, Y. (1998), The role of ease of use, usefulness and attitude in the prediction of World Wide Web usage, Proceedings of the 1998 Association for Computing Machinery Special Interest Group on Computer Personnel Research.

[2] Succi, M.J., Walter, Z.D. (1999). Theory of user acceptance of information technologies: An examination of health care professionals, 32nd Hawaii International Conference on System Sciences, Hawaii, IEEE Computer Society.

[3] Pikkarainen,T., Pikkarainen,K.,Karjaluoto,H.,Pahnila.S.,(2004), Consumer acceptance of online banking: an extension of the technology acceptance model, 14(3), Internet research, 224–235 www.emeralinsight.con/researchregister.

[4] Mathieson, K. (1991). Predicting User Intentions: Comparing the Technology Acceptance Model with the Theory of Planned Behavior, Information Systems Research, 2(3), 173-191.

[5] Obstfelder, A., Engeseth, K.H., Wynn, R., (2007).Characteristics of successfully implemented telemedical applications, Implement Sci. 2 (25). Aggelidis, V. P., Chatzoglou, P. D. (2009). Using a modified technology acceptance model in hospitals, International Journal of Medical Informatics, 78(2), 115-126.

[6] Tung, F.C., Chang, S.C., Chou, C.M. (2008). An extension of trust and TAM model with IDT in the adoption of the electronic logistics information system in HIS in the medical industry, Int. J. Med. Inform. 77 (5), 324–335.

[7] Walter, Z., Lopez M.S.(2008). Physicians acceptance of information technology: Role of perceived threat to professional autonomy, Decision Support Systems, 46(1), 206-215.

[8] Kijsanayotin, B., Pannarunothai, S., Speedie, S.M., (2009), Factors influencing health information technology adoption in Thailand's community health centers: Applying the UTAUT model, International Journal Medical Informatics, 79, 404-416.

[9] Gagnon, M.P, Pluye, P., Desmartis, M., Car, J., Pagliari, C., Labrecque, M., Fremont, P., Gagnon, J., Nojya, M., Legare, F. (2010), A systematic review of interventions promoting clinical information retrieval technology (CIRT) adoption by healthcare professionals, International Journal of Medical Informatics, 79, 669-680.

[10] Van Bemmel, J. H., Musen, M. A. (1997). Handbook of medical informatics. NY: Springer.

[11] Chang, I-C., Hwang, H-G., Hung, W-F., Li, Y-C., (2007), Physicians' acceptance of pharmacokinetics-based clinical decision support systems, Expert Systems with Applications, 33, (2), 296–303.

[12] Paul, D.L., McDaniel, R.R., Jr. (2004). A field study of the effect of interpersonal trust on virtual collaborative relationship performance, MIS Quarterly 28 (2), 183–227.

[13] Schaper, L.K., Pervan, G.P (2007). ICT and OTs: a model of information and communication technology acceptance and utilization by occupational therapists, International Journal of Medical Informatics, 76, 212-221.

[14] Dowswell, G. Harrison, S. Wright, J. (2001). Clinical guidelines: attitudes, information processes and culture in English primary care, International Journal of Health Planning and Management, 16 (2), 107–124.

[15] Goldman, L. (1974). Doctors' attitudes toward national health insurance. Medical Care, 12 (5), 413–423.

[16] Harrington, C., (1975). Medical ideologies in conflict. Medical Care, 13(11) 905 –914.

[17] Hayward, R.S.A., Moore, K.A. (1997).Canadian physicians' attitudes about and preferences regarding clinical practice guidelines, Canadian Medical Association Journal, 156 (12) 1715–1723.

[18] Borkowski, N.M., Allen, W.R. (2003). Does attribution theory explain physicians' nonacceptance of clinical practice guidelines?, Hospital Topics: Research and Perspectives on Healthcare, 81 (2), 9–21.

[19] Larson, M.S. (1977). The Rise of professionalism: A sociological analysis, University of California Press, Berkeley, CA.

[20] Sharma, A. (1997), Professionals as agent: knowledge asymmetry in agency exchanges, Academy of Management Review, 22 (3),758–798.

[21] Watts, C.(2008). Erosion of healthcare professional autonomy and public respect for the profession. Surgical Neurology, 71(3), 269-273.

[22] Raelin, J. (1989). An anatomy of autonomy: managing professionals, The Academy of Management Executive, 3 (3), 216–228.

[23] Smith, D.H., Pettegrew L. S. (1986), Mutual persuasion as a model for doctor-patient communication, Theoretical Medicine, 7(2), 127-146.

[24] Magne, N., Olaf, A. (2007), Doctors' learning habits: CME activities among Norwegian physicians over the last decade, BMC Medical Education, 7(1), 10.

[25] Chau, P.Y.K., Hu, P.J. (2002).Investigating healthcare professionals' decision to accept telemedicine technology: an empirical test of competing theories, Information and Management 39 (4), 297–311

[26] Zuger A. (2004). Dissatisfaction with medical practice. N Engl J Med, 350 (1),69-75.

[27] Montague, E.N.H., Kleiner B.M. Winchester W.W. (2009). Empirically understanding trust in medical technology. International Journal of Industrial Ergonomics, 39 (4), 628-634.

[28] Starr P. (1982). The second transformation of American medicine. New York: Basic Books, Inc.

[29] Abbott, A. (1988). The System of Professions: An Essay on the Division of Expert Labor, University of Chicago Press, Chicago, IL.

[30] Adams, D.W. (1980). Standards and the development of professions: Implications for educational evaluation. Paper presented at the 64th Annual Meeting of the American Educational Research Association. http://eric.ed.gov/ERICWebPortal/custom/portlets/recordDetails/detailmini.jsp?_nfpb=true&_&ERICExtSearch_SearchValue_0=ED193291&ERICExtSearch_SearchType_0=eric_acc_no& accno=ED193291(Accessed October 16, 2011)
[31] Lengermann, J.J.(1971), Supposed and actual differences in professional autonomy among CPAs as related to type of work organization and size of firm, The Accounting Review, 46 (4), 665–675.
[32] Freidson, E. (1970), Professional Dominance: The Social Structure of Medicine, Atherton Press, New York.
[33] Freidson, E. (1988). Profession of Medicine: A Study of the Sociology of Applied Knowledge, The University of Chicago Press, Chicago, IL.
[34] Schainblatt, A.H. (1982), How companies measure the productivity of engineers and scientists, Research Management 25(3), 10–18.
[35] Wilson, D.K., Mueser, R. , Raelin, J.A. (1994). New look at performance appraisal for scientists and engineers, Research Technology Management. 37(4), 51–55.
[36] Bonora, E.A, Revang, O.(1991). A strategic framework for analyzing professional service firm _ developing strategies for sustained performance, Strategic Management Society Inter organizational Conference, Toronto, Canada
[37] Nonaka, I.,Takeuchi, H.(1995). The knowledge –creating company, Oxford University Press, New York.
[38] Harrison, S. Dowswell, G., Wright, J. (2002). Practice nurses and clinical guidelines in a changing primary care context: an empirical study, Journal of advanced nursing, 39 (3), 299–307.
[39] Lowenhaupt, M. (2004). Removing barriers to technology. The Physician Executive, 30(2), 12-14.
[40] Bucy, E. P. (2004). The interactivity paradox: Closer to the news but confused. In Media access: Social and psychological dimensions of new technology use, eds. E. P. Bucy and J. E. Newhagen, pp. 47–72. Mahwah, NJ: Lawrence Erlbaum Associates.
[41] Zack, M. H. (1993). Interactivity and communication mode choices in ongoing management groups. Information System Research, 4(3), 207–239.
[42] McMillan, S. J., and Hwang, J-S. (2002). Measures of perceived interactivity: An exploration of the role of direction of communication, user control, and time in shaping perceptions of interactivity. Journal of Advertising 31(3):29–42
[43] McMillan, S. J. (2002). Exploring models of interactivity from multiple research traditions: Users, documents, and systems. In Handbook of new media, eds. L. Lievrouw and S. Livingston, pp. 163–182. London: Sage.
[44] Rafaeli, S., Sudweeks, F. (1998). Interactivity on the Nets. In Network and netplay: Virtual groups on the Internet, eds. F. Sudweeks, M. McLaughlin, and S. Rafaeli, pp. 173–189. Menlo Park, CA: AAAI Press/MIT Press.

[45] Steuer, J. (1995). Defining virtual reality: Dimensions determining telepresence. In Communication in the age of virtual reality, eds. F. Biocca and M. R. Levy, (pp. 33–56). Hillsdale, NJ: Lawrence Erlbaum Associates.

[46] Neuman, W. R. (1991). The future of the mass audience. New York: Cambridge University Press.

[47] Williams, F., Rice, R. E., Rogers, E. M. (1988). Research methods and the new media. New York: Free Press.

[48] Jensen, J. F. (1998). Interactivity: Tracking a new concept in media and communication studies. Nordicom Review 1:185–204.

[49] Reeves, B., Nass, C. (1996). The Media Equation: How People Treat Computers, Television, and New Media Like Real People and Places, New York: Cambridge University Press/CSLI.

[50] Stromer-Galley, J. (2000). Online interaction and why candidates avoid it. Journal of Communication 50(4):111–132.

[51] Rafaeli, S. (1988). Interactivity: From new media to communication. In Advancing communication science: Merging mass and interpersonal processes, eds. R. Hawkins, J. Wiemann, and S. Pingree, (pp. 110– 134). Newbury Park, CA: Sage.

[52] Massey, B. L., and Levy, M. R. (1999). Interactivity, online journalism, and English-languageWeb newspapers in Asia. Journalism & Mass Communication Quarterly 76(1):138–151.

Burgoon, J. K., Bonito, J. A., Bengtsson, B., Cederberg, C., Lundeberg, M., Allspach, L. (2000). Interactivity in human-computer interaction: interaction: A study of credibility, understanding, and influence. Computers in Human Behavior 16,553–574.

[53] Hanssen, L., Jankowski, N.W., Etienne R (1996), Interactivity from the Perspective of Communication Studies," in Contours of Multimedia: Recent Technological, Theoretical, and Empirical Developments, N.W. Jankowski and L. Hanssen, eds., Luton, UK: University of Luton Press, 61-73,

[54] Moon, Y., Nass, C. (1996). How 'Real' Are Computer Personalities? Psychological Responses to Personality Types in Human-Computer Interaction. Communication Research, 2Z (6), 651-614.

[55] Sundar, S. S., Nass, C.(2000), Source Orientation in Human-Computer Interaction: Programmer, Networker, or Independent Social Actor?, Communication Research, 27 (6), 683-703.

[56] Berthon, P., Pitt, L., Watson, R.T.(1996), Marketing communication and the worldwide web. Business Horizons, 39(5), 24-32.

[57] Coyle, J.R., Thorson, E. (2001). The Effects of Progressive Levels of Interactivity and Vividness in Web Marketing Sites, Journal of Advertising. 30 (3), 65-77.

[58] Bucy, E.P. (2003). Media credibility reconsidered: Synergy effects between on-air and online news. Journalism and Mass Communication Quarterly, 80(2),247-264.

[59] Kalyanaraman, S., Sundar, S.S., (2003). The Psychological Appeal of Personalized Online Content: An Experimental Investigation of Customized Web Portals, Paper presented at the meeting of the International Communication Association, San Diego, May.

[60] Fogg, B. J. (2003). Persuasive Technology: Using Computers to Change What We Think and Do. Boston: Morgan Kaufmann.

[61] Agarwal, R., .Karahanna, E., (2000). Time Flies when You're Having Fun: Cognitive Absorption and Beliefs about Information Technology Usage. MIS Quarterly, 24, 665-694.

[62] Nonaka, I.,Takeuchi, H.(1995). The knowledge –creating company, Oxford University Press, New York.Varonen H, Kortteisto T, Kaila M, for the EBMeDS Study Group (2008). What may help or hinder the implementation of computerized decision support systems (CDSSs): a focus group study with physicians. Fam Pract, 2;25(3):162-7.

[63] Sittig D, Krall M, Dykstra R, et al. (2006), A survey of factors affecting clinician acceptance of clinical decision support. BMC Med Inform Decis Mak , 6(1):6.

[64] Pain, D., Fielden, K., Shibl, R.A. (2003), Options on the use of clinical decision support systems for paediatric prescribing in a New Zealand hospital, Logistics Information Management, 16(¾) 201-206.

[65] Mclaughlin, J., Webster, A. (1998), Rationalizing knowledge: IT systems, professional identifies and power, The Sociological Review, 46 (4),781–802.

[66] Kleiner,B.M., (2006), Sociotechnical system design in health care. In: Carayon, P. (ED.), Handbook of Human Factors and Ergonomics in Health Care and Patient Safety, Lawrence Erbaum Associates INC., Mahwah. 79 94.

[67] Lacramioara, S. Vasile, S. (2006), Human_computer interaction reflected in the design of user interfaces for general practitioner, Int. J.Med. Inform. 75, 335-342.

[68] Osheroff, JA. (2009). Improving medication use and outcomes with clinical decision support: a step-by-step guide. Chicago, IL: The Healthcare Information and Management Systems Society.

[69] Berner, ES. (2009). Clinical decision support systems: State of the Art. AHRQ Publication No.09-0069-EF. Rockville, Maryland: Agency for Healthcare Research and Quality.

[70] Miller RA, Waitman LR, Chen S, et al. (2005). The anatomy of decision support during inpatient care provider order entry (CPOE): empirical observations from a decade of CPOE experience at Vanderbilt. J Biomed Inform , 38(6):469-85.

[71] McMillan, S. J., and Hwang, J-S. (2002). Measures of perceived interactivity: An exploration of the role of direction of communication, user control, and time in shaping perceptions of interactivity. Journal of Advertising 31(3):29–42

[72] Pianesi, F., Graziola, I., Zancanaro, M., Goren-Bar, D., (2009). The Motivational and Control Structure Underlying the Acceptance of Adaptive Museum Guides - An Empirical Study, Interacting with Computers, 21(3), 186-200.

[73] Hoffman, D. L., Novak, T. P., (1996). Marketing in Hypermedia Computer Mediated Environemnts: Conceptual Foundations. Journal of Marketing, 60, 50-68.

[74] Prasad, P., Prasad, A. (1994). The ideology of professionalism and work computerization: institutionalist study of technological change, Human Relations,47 (12), 1433–1458.

Chapter 3

Supporting E-Health Information Seekers: From Simple Strategies to Knowledge-Based Methods

Lina F. Soualmia, Badisse Dahamna and Stéfan J. Darmoni

Additional information is available at the end of the chapter

http://dx.doi.org/10.5772/50348

1. Introduction

Today, a web search is clearly one of the foremost methods for finding information. The growth of the Internet and the increasing availability of online resources have made the task of searching a crucial one. However, searching the web is not always as successful as users expect it to be and Internet users have to make a great effort to formulate a search query that returns the required results. Information retrieval concentrates on developing algorithms to locate and select documents from a corpus that are relevant to a given query. The development of online information retrieval tools, such as search engines or search robots many of which utilize hyperlink analysis [1], has been greatly beneficial to Internet users [2]. In the health domain, users are now experiencing huge difficulties in finding precisely what they are looking for among the numerous documents available online, and this in spite of existing tools. In medicine and health-related information accessible on the Internet, general search engines, such as Google, or general catalogues, such as Yahoo, cannot solve this problem efficiently [3]. This is because they usually offer a selection of documents that turn out to be either too large or ill-suited to the query. Free text word-based search engines typically return innumerable completely irrelevant hits, which require much manual weeding by the user, and also miss important information resources.

In this context, several health gateways [4] have been developed to support systematic resource discovery and help users find the health information they are looking for. These information seekers may be patients but also health professionals, such as physicians searching for clinical trials. Health gateways rely on thesauri and controlled vocabularies. Some of them are evaluated in [5]. Medical thesauri are a proven key technology for effective access to health information since they provide a controlled vocabulary for indexing documents and coding electronic health records. They therefore help to overcome some of the problems of free-text search by linking and grouping terms and concepts.

Nonetheless, medical vocabularies are difficult to handle by non-professionals. Problems also arise because there are practically as many different terminologies, controlled vocabularies, thesauri and classification systems as there are fields of application in health. We give in this chapter a panel of techniques that may be applied to help health information seekers. All the tests are performed on the CISMeF catalogue (Catalogue and Index of Medical Sites in French) [6] but are reproducible in other languages and other medical applications.

The remainder of the chapter is organized as follows: in section 2 we start by describing the CISMeF catalogue. The section 3 is devoted to simple search techniques such as approximate string matching and heuristics for queries composed by several words. Another method consists in meta-modeling health terminologies to improve information retrieval, the description of which is in the section 4. In the section 5 we describe the data-mining process to extract new knowledge and relations between terms to allow users to extend their searches.

2. The CISMeF catalogue

The CISMeF project was initiated in February 1995. As opposed to Yahoo, CISMeF is cataloguing the most important and quality-controlled sources of institutional health information in French. The CISMeF catalogue describes and indexes a large number of health-information resources of high quality (n=13,452 in October 2003; n=90,056 in May 2012). A resource can be a web site, web pages, documents, reports and teaching material: any support that may contain health information.

CISMeF takes into account the diversity of the end-users and allow them to find good quality resources. These resources are selected according to strict criteria by a team of librarians and are indexed according to a methodology which involves a four-fold process: resource collection, filtering, description and indexing. CISMeF is a quality-controlled gateway such as defined by Koch [4]. The following elements that characterize a typical quality-controlled health gateway are fulfilled in CISMeF: selection and collection development, collection management, intellectual creation of metadata, resource description (a metadata set), resource indexing (with controlled vocabulary system). To include only reliable resources, and to assess the quality of health information on the Internet, the main criteria (*e.g.* source, description, disclosure, last update) of CISMeF are from HONCode[1]. In the following sections we describe the set of metadata elements and the reference dictionary used in the catalogue.

2.1. CISMeF metadata

The notion of metadata was around before the Internet but its importance has grown with the increasing number of electronic publications and digital libraries. The World Wide Web Consortium (W3C) have proposed that metadata should be used to describe the data

[1] http://www.hon.ch/

contained on the web and to add semantic markup to web resources, thus describing their content and functionalities, from the vocabulary defined in terminologies and ontologies.

Metadata are data about data, and in the web context, these are data describing web resources. When properly implemented, metadata enhance information retrieval. The CISMeF uses several sets of metadata. Among them there is the Dublin Core (DC) [7] metadata set, which is a 15-element set intended to aid discovery of electronic resources. The resources indexed in CISMeF are described by eleven of the Dublin Core elements: *author, date, description, format, identifier, language, editor, type of resource, rights, subject* and *title.* DC is not a complete solution; it cannot be used to describe the quality or location of a resource. To fill these gaps, CISMeF uses its own elements to extend the DC standard. Eight elements are specific to CISMeF: *institution, city, province, country, target public, access type, sponsorships,* and *cost.* The user type is also taken into account. The CISMeF have defined two additional fields for resources intended for health professionals: indication of the *evidence-based medicine,* and the *method* used to determine it. For teaching resources, eleven elements of the IEEE 1484 LOM (Learning Object Metadata) "Educational" category are added.

2.2. CISMeF controlled vocabulary

Thesauri are a proven key technology for effective access to information as they provide a controlled vocabulary for indexing information. They therefore help to overcome some of the problems of free-text search by relating and grouping relevant terms in a specific domain. The main thesaurus used for medical information is the Medical Subject Headings (MeSH) [8] thesaurus used by the U.S. National Library of Medicine to index MEDLINE articles. The core of MeSH is a hierarchical structure that consists of sets of descriptors. At the top level we find general headings (*e.g.* diseases), and at deeper levels we find more specific headings (*e.g.* asthma). The 2012 version of the MeSH contains over 26,581 main headings (*e.g.* hepatitis, abdomen) and 83 subheadings (*e.g.* diagnosis, complications). Together with a main heading, a subheading allows to specify which particular aspect of the main heading is being addressed. For example, the pair [hepatitis/diagnosis] specifies the diagnosis aspect of hepatitis. For each main heading, MeSH defines a subset of allowable qualifiers so that only certain pairs can be used as indexing terms (*e.g.* aphasia/metabolism and hand/surgery are allowable, but hand/metabolism is not). The reference dictionary of CISMeF (the structure of which is detailed in Table 1) was created between 1995 and 2005 exclusively on the French version of the MeSH thesaurus maintained by the US National Library of Medicine, completed by numerous synonyms in French collected by the CISMeF team.

Several add-ons were performed around the MeSH thesaurus to index Web resources instead of scientific articles [9]: super-concepts (or Meta-terms) to optimize information retrieval and categorization, and resource types (organized hierarchically since 1997 *vs.* MeSH publication types' hierarchy since 2006). Indeed, MeSH main headings and subheadings are organized hierarchically but these hierarchies do not allow a complete view concerning a specialty. The main headings and subheadings in the CISMeF controlled vocabulary are brought together under metaterms (*e.g.* cardiology). Metaterms (n=73) concern medical specialties and it is possible by browsing to know sets of MeSH main headings and subheadings qualifiers which are semantically related to the same specialty but dispersed in several trees. The MeSH thesaurus was originally used to index biomedical scientific articles for the MEDLINE database. In addition to the set of metaterms, the CISMeF team has modeled a hierarchy of resource types (n=127), to customize MeSH to the field of e-health resources. These resource types describe the nature of the resource (*e.g.* teaching material, clinical guidelines, patient forums), and are a generalization or extension of the MEDLINE publication types. Each resource in CISMeF is described with a set of MeSH main headings, subheadings and CISMeF resource types. Each main heading, [main heading/subheading] pair, and resource type is allotted a 'minor' or 'major' weight, according to the importance of the concept it refers to in the resource. Major terms are marked by a star (*).

	MeSH Terms	MeSH Synonyms	CISMeF synonyms	Total
1 word	9,679	9,391	3,359	22,429
2 words	9,833	28,051	8,258	46,142
3 words	4,204	19,551	6,569	30,324
4 words and +	2,503	16,992	4,924	24,419

Table 1. Composition of the reference dictionary based on the MeSH in French.

2.3. Searching through the catalogue

Many ways of navigation and information retrieval are possible in the catalogue [6]. The most used is the simple search (free text interface). It is based on subsumption relationships. If the query can be matched with an existing term of the terminology, thus the result is the union of the resources that are indexed by the term, and the resources that are indexed by the terms it subsumes, directly or indirectly, in all the hierarchies it belongs to. If the query cannot be matched, the search is done over the other fields of the metadata and in a worse case a full-text search is carried out. Contrary to MEDLINE, the resource types and the meta-terms were voluntary made ambiguous to maximize the recall (e.g. in the query guidelines in virology, virology will be recognized as a meta-term (instead of a term) and guidelines will be recognized as both the term and the resource type because we assume most of end users confuse content and container). In the following section we propose some simple enhancements for health information seekers' queries matching.

3. Spell-checking queries

A simple spelling corrector, such as Google's "*Did you mean:*" or Yahoo's "*Also try:*" feature may be a valuable tool for non-professional users who may approach the medical domain in a more general way [10]. Such features can improve the performance of these tools and provide the user with the necessary help. In fact, the problem of spelling errors represents a major challenge for an information retrieval system. If the queries (composed by one or multiple words) generated by information seekers remain undetected, this can result in a lack of outcome in terms of search and retrieval. A spelling corrector may be classified in two categories. The first relies on a dictionary of well-spelled terms and selects the top candidate based on a string edit distance calculus. An approximate string matching algorithm, or a function, is required to detect errors in users' queries. It then recommends a list of terms, from the reference dictionary, that are similar to each query word. The second category of spelling correctors uses lexical disambiguation tools in order to refine the ranking of the candidate terms that might be a correction of the misspelled query.

3.1. Related work

Several studies have been published on this subject. We cite the work of Grannis [11] which describes a method for calculating similarity in order to improve medical record linkage. This method uses different algorithms such as Jaro-Winkler, Levenshtein [12] and the longest common subsequence (LCS). In [13] the authors suggest improving the algorithm for computing Levenshtein similarity by using the frequency and length of strings. In [14] a phonetic transcription corrects users' queries when they are misspelled but have similar pronunciation (*e.g.* Alzaymer *vs.* Alzheimer). In [15] the authors propose a simple and flexible spell-checker using efficient associative matching in a neural system and also compare their method with other commonly used spell-checkers. In fact, the problem of automatic spell checking is not new. Indeed, research in this area started in the 1960's [16] and many different techniques for spell-checking have been proposed since then. Some of those techniques exploit general spelling error tendencies and others exploit phonetic transcription of the misspelled term to find the correct term. The process of spell-checking can generally be divided into three steps:

i. error detection: the validity of a term in a language is verified and invalid terms are identified as spelling errors;
ii. error correction: valid candidate terms from the dictionary are selected as corrections for the misspelled term;
iii. ranking: the selected corrections are sorted in decreasing order of their likelihood of being the intended term.

Many studies have been performed to analyze the types and the tendencies of spelling errors for the English language. According to [17] spelling errors are generally divided into two types, (i) typographic errors and (ii) cognitive errors. Typographic errors occur when the correct spelling is known but the word is mistyped by mistake. These errors are mostly related to keyboard errors and therefore do not follow any linguistic criteria (58% of these errors involve adjacent keys [18] and occur because the wrong key is pressed, or two keys are pressed, or keys are pressed in the wrong order …*etc.*). Cognitive errors, or orthographic errors, occur when the correct spelling of a term is not known. The pronunciation of the misspelled term is similar to the pronunciation of the intended correct term. In English, the role of the sound similarity of characters is a factor that often affects error tendencies [18]. However, phonetic errors are harder to correct because they deform the word more than a single insertion, deletion or substitution. Damereau [16] indicated that 80% of all spelling errors fall into one of the following four single edit operation categories : (i) transposition of two adjacent letters (*ashtma* vs. *asthma*) (ii) insertion of one letter (*asthmma* vs. *asthma*) (iii) deletion of one letter (*astma* vs. *asthma*) and (iv) replacement of one letter by another (*asthla* vs. *asthma*). Each of these wrong operations costs 1 *i.e.* the distance between the misspelled and the correct word [[17].

The third step in spell-checking is the ranking of the selected corrections. Main spell-checking techniques do not provide any explicit mechanism. However, statistical techniques [19] provide ranking of the corrections based on probability scores [20] with good results [21]. HONselect [22] is a multilingual and intelligent search tool integrating heterogeneous web resources in health. In the medical domain, spell-checking is performed on the basis of a medical thesaurus by offering information seekers several medical terms, ranging from one to four differences related to the original query. Exploiting the frequency of a given term in the medical domain can also significantly improve spelling correction [23]: edit distance technique is used for correction along with term frequencies for ranking. In [24] the authors use normalization techniques, aggressive reformatting and abbreviation expansion for unrecognized words as well as spelling correction to find the closest drug names within RxNorm for drug name variants that can be found in local drug formularies. It returns only drug name suggestions. To match queries with the MeSH thesaurus, Wilbur et al. [25] proposed a technique on the noisy channel model and statistics from the PubMed logs.

3.2. Proposed method

Research has focused on several different areas, from pattern matching algorithms and dictionary searching techniques to optical character recognition of spelling corrections in different domains. However, the literature is quite sparse in the medical domain, which is a distinct problem, because of the complexity of medical vocabularies. In this section, a simple method is proposed: it combines two approximate string comparators, the well-known Levenshtein [6] edit distance and the Stoilos function similarity defined in [26] for ontologies. We apply and evaluate these two distances, alone and combined, on a set of sample queries in French submitted to the health gateway CISMeF. A set of 127,750 queries were extracted from the query log server (3 months logs). Only the most frequent queries were selected. In fact some queries are more frequent than others. For example, the query *"swine flu"* is more present in the query log than *"chlorophyll"*. We eliminated the doubles (68,712 queries remained). From these 68,712 queries, we selected 25,000 queries to extract those with no answers (7,562). A set of 6,297 frequent queries was constituted from the original set of 7,562 by eliminating those that were submitted only once. In this set, the queries were composed from 1 to 4 and more words as detailed in the Table 2.

Composition	Number
1 word	1,061
2 words	1,636
3 words	1,443
4 (and more) words	2,157
Total	6,297

Table 2. Structure of the queries (with no answer) obtained from the logs.

3.2.1. Similarity functions

Similarity functions between two text strings S_1 and S_2 give a similarity or dissimilarity score between S_1 and S_2 for approximate matching or comparison. For example, the strings "*Asthma*" and "*Asthmatic*" can be considered similar to a certain degree. Modern spell-checking tools are based on the simple Levenshtein edit distance [12] which is the most widely known. This function operates between two input strings and returns a score equivalent to the number of substitutions and deletions needed in order to transform one input string into another. It is defined as the minimum number of elementary operations that is required to pass from a string S_1 to a string S_2. There are three possible transactions: replacing a character with another, deleting a character and adding a character. This measure takes its values in the interval [0, ∞ [. The Normalized Levenshtein [27] (*LevNorm*) in the range [0,1] is obtained by dividing the distance of Levenshtein $Lev(S_1, S_2)$ by the size of the longest string and it is defined by the following equation ():

$$\text{LevNorm}(S_1,S_2)=\frac{\text{Lev }(S_1,S_2)}{\text{Max}(|S_1|,|S_2|)} \tag{1}$$

For example, LevNorm(eutanasia, euthanasia)=0.1, as Lev(eutanasia, eut**h**anasia)=1 (adds 1 character h); |eutanasia|=9 and |euthanasia|=10.

We complete the calculation of the Levenshtein distance by the similarity function Stoilos proposed in [26]. It has been specifically developed for strings that are labels of concepts in ontologies. It is based on the idea that the similarity between two entities is related to their commonalities as well as their differences. Thus, the similarity should be a function of both these features. It is defined by the equation (2) where $Comm(S_1,S_2)$ stands for the commonality between the strings S_1 and S_2, $Diff(S_1,S_2)$ for the difference between S_1 and S_2, and $Winkler(S_1,S_2)$ for the improvement of the result using the method introduced by Winkler in [28]:

$$\text{Sim}\left(S_{1,}S_2\right)=Comm\left(S_{1,}S_2\right)-Diff\left(S_{1,}S_2\right)+winkler\left(S_{1,}S_2\right) \tag{2}$$

The function of commonality is determined by the substring function. The biggest common substring between two strings (*MaxComSubString*) is computed. This process is further extended by removing the common substring and by searching again for the next biggest substring until none can be identified. The function of commonality is given by the equation (3):

$$\text{Comm}\left(S_1,S_2\right)=\frac{2\times\sum_i|\text{MaxComSubString}_i|}{|S_1|+|S_2|} \tag{3}$$

For example, for S_1=**Trigonocepa**hl**ie** and S_2=**Trigonocep**ha**lie** we have: |MaxComSubString_1| = |Trigonocep|=10, |MaxComSubString_2| =|lie|=3 and *Comm*(Trigonocepahlie,Trigonocephalie) = 0.866.

The difference function *Diff(S1,S2)* is based on the length of the unmatched strings resulting from the initial matching step. The function of difference is defined in equation (4) where $p \in [0, \infty[$, $|u_{S1}|$ and $|u_{S2}|$ represent the length of the unmatched substring from the strings S_1 and S_2 scaled respectively by their length :

$$\text{Diff}(S_1,S_2) = \frac{|u_{S1}| \times |u_{S2}|}{p + (1-p) \times (|u_{S1}| + |u_{S2}| - |u_{S1}| \times |u_{S2}|)} \quad (4)$$

For example for S1=Trigonocepahlie and S2=Trigonocephalie and p=0.6 we have: $|u_{S1}|$ = 2/15; $|u_{S2}|$ =2/15; *Diff(S1,S2)* =0.0254.

The Winkler parameter *Winkler(S1,S2)* is a factor that improves the results. It is defined by the equation (5) where *L* is the length of common prefix between the strings S_1 and S_2 at the start of the string up to a maximum of 4 characters and *P* is a constant scaling factor for how much the score is adjusted upwards for having common prefixes. The standard value for this constant in Winkler's work is *P=0.1* :

$$\text{Winkler}(S_1,S_2) = L \times P \times (1 - Comm(S_1,S_2)) \quad (5)$$

For example, for between S1=hyperaldoterisme and S2=hyperaldosteronisme, we have |S1|=16, |S2|=19; the common substrings between S1 and S2 are hyperaldo, ter, and isme. Comm(S1,S2)=0.914; Diff(S1,S2)=0; Winkler(S1,S2)=0.034 and Sim(**hyperaldoterisme,hyper aldoster**onisme)=0.948.

3.2.2. Processing users' queries

As detailed in [18], spelling errors can be classified as typographic and phonetic. Cognitive errors are caused by a writer's lack of knowledge and phonetic ones are due to similar pronunciation of a misspelled and corrected word. We pre-process the queries by a phonetic transcription with the algorithm described in [14]. To process multi-word queries, we used the following basic natural language processing steps and the well-known Bag-of-Words (BoW) algorithm before applying similarity functions:

1. *Query segmentation*: the query was segmented in words thanks to a list of segmentation characters and *string tokenizers*. This list is composed of all the non-alphanumerical characters (*e.g.*: * $,!§;|@).
2. *Character normalizations*: we applied two types of character normalization at this stage. MeSH terms are in the form of non-accented uppercase characters. Nevertheless, the terms used in the CISMeF terminology are in mixed-case and accented. (1) *Lowercase conversion*: all the uppercased characters were replaced by their lowercase version; *"A"* was replaced by *"a"*. This step was necessary because the controlled vocabulary is in lowercase. (2) *Deaccenting*: all accented characters (*"éèêë"*) were replaced by non-accented (*"e"*) ones. Words in the French MeSH were not accented, and words in queries were either accented or not, or wrongly accented (*hèpatite"* instead *"hépatite"*).

3. *Stop words*: we eliminated all stop words (such as *the, and, when*) in the query. Our stop word list was composed 1,422 elements in French (*vs.* 135 in PubMed).
4. *Exact match expression*: we use regular expressions to match the exact expression of each word of the query with the terminology. This step allowed us to take into account the complex terms (composed of more than one word) of the reference dictionary and also to avoid some inherent noise generated by the truncations. The query *'**accident**'* is matched with the term *'circulation **accident**'* but not with the terms *'**accident**s'* and *'chute **accident**elle'*. The query *'**sida**'* is matched with the terms *'lymphome lié **sida**'* and *'**sida** atteinte neurologique'* but not with the terms *'gluco**sida**ses'*, *'agra**sida**e'* and *'bêta galacto**sida**se'* which are not relevant.
5. *Phonemisation:* It converts a word into its French phonemic transcription: *e.g.* the query *alzaymer* is replaced by the reserved term *alzheimer*.
6. *Bag of words:* The algorithm searched the greatest set of words in the query corresponding to a reserved term. The query was segmented. The stop words were eliminated. The other words were transformed with the *Phonemisation* function and sorted alphabetically. The different reserved term bags were formed iteratively until there were no possible combinations. The query *'therapy of the breast cancer'* gave two reserved words: *'therapeutics'* and *'breast cancer'* (*therapy* being a synonym of the reserved term *therapeutics).*

3.2.3. Evaluations

To evaluate our method of correcting misspellings, we used the standard measures of evaluation of information retrieval systems, by calculating precision, recall and the F-Measure. We performed a manual evaluation to determine these measures. Precision (6) measured the proportion of queries that were properly corrected among those corrected.

$$Precision = \frac{|\{Queries\ correctly\ corrected\}|}{|\{Queries\ corrected\}|} \tag{6}$$

Recall (7) measured the proportion of queries that were properly corrected among those requiring correction.

$$Recall = \frac{|\{Queries\ correctly\ corrected\}|}{|\{Queries\ to\ be\ corrected\}|} \tag{7}$$

The F-Measure combined the precision and recall by the following equation (8) :

$$F - Measure = \frac{2 \times Precision \times Recall}{(Precision + Recall)} \tag{8}$$

We also calculated confidence intervals at ρ=5% to avoid evaluating the whole set of queries, but some sets that are manually manageable. For a proportion x and a set of size n_x the confidence interval is:

$$CI_x = \left[x - 1.96 \times \sqrt{\frac{x \times (1-x)}{n_x}} ; x + 1.96 \times \sqrt{\frac{x \times (1-x)}{n_x}} \right] \quad (9)$$

3.2.4. Results

The Levenshtein and Stoilos functions require a choice of thresholds to obtain a manageable number of correction suggestions for the user. We tested, in a previous work, different thresholds [29] for the normalized Levenshtein distance, the similarity function of Stoilos and for the combination of both on a set of 163 queries. The best results were obtained with Levenshtein>0.2 and Stoilos>0.7. To determine the impact of the size of the query we measured the number of suggestions of corrected queries (on the set of 6,297 frequent queries) in the Table 3. For a user, the maximum number of manageable suggestions for one query was 6.

	Nb characters	Nb suggestions by query
1 word query	Min = 3; Avg = 10.49 ; Max = 25	Avg = 0.39 ; Max = 5
2 words query	Min = 5; Avg = 18.36; Max = 41	Avg = 0.22 ; Max = 6
3 words query	Min = 10; Avg = 24.39; Max = 54	Avg = 0.13; Max = 1
4 words and +query	Min = 11; Avg = 37.30; Max = 113	Avg = 0.06; Max = 1

Table 3. Number of suggestions according to the size of the queries.

Manual evaluations were performed on sets of ~1/3 of each type of queries. Evaluations of the quality of queries suggestions (Precision, Recall and F-Measure) were performed manually on several sets, according to the size of the query, but also according to the following methods : Bag-of-Words, Levenshtein distance alongside the Stoilos similarity function, but also the Bag-of-Words processed before and after the combination of the Levenshtein distance along with the Stoilos similarity function. Levenshtein and Stoilos remained constant at <0.2 and >0.7 respectively. The resulting curves are in Figures 1, 2 and 3. By combining the Bag-of-Words algorithm along with the Levenshtein distance and the similarity function of Stoilos, a total of 1,418 (22.52 %) queries matched medical terms or combinations of medical terms. The remaining queries with no suggestions (when terms and also the possible combination of terms) not belong to the dictionary. For 1-word queries, it remained 711 (67%), for 2-words queries it remained 1197 queries (73.16%); for 3-words queries it remained 1126 (78.08%) and for 4 words queries it remained 1,846 queries (85.58%). For example, the query "*nutrithérapie*" (nutritherapy) contains no error but cannot be matched with any medical term in the reference dictionary. Evaluations shown that best results were obtained by performing the Bag-of-Words algorithm before the combination of Levenshtein alongside Stoilos.

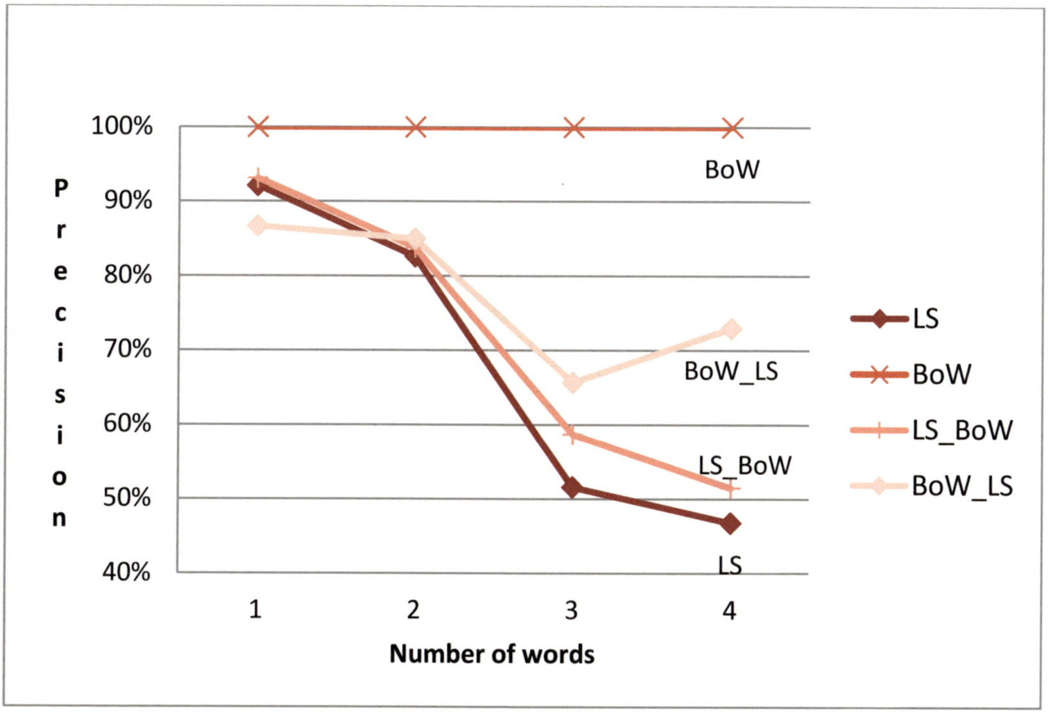

Figure 1. Precision curves according to the size of the query.

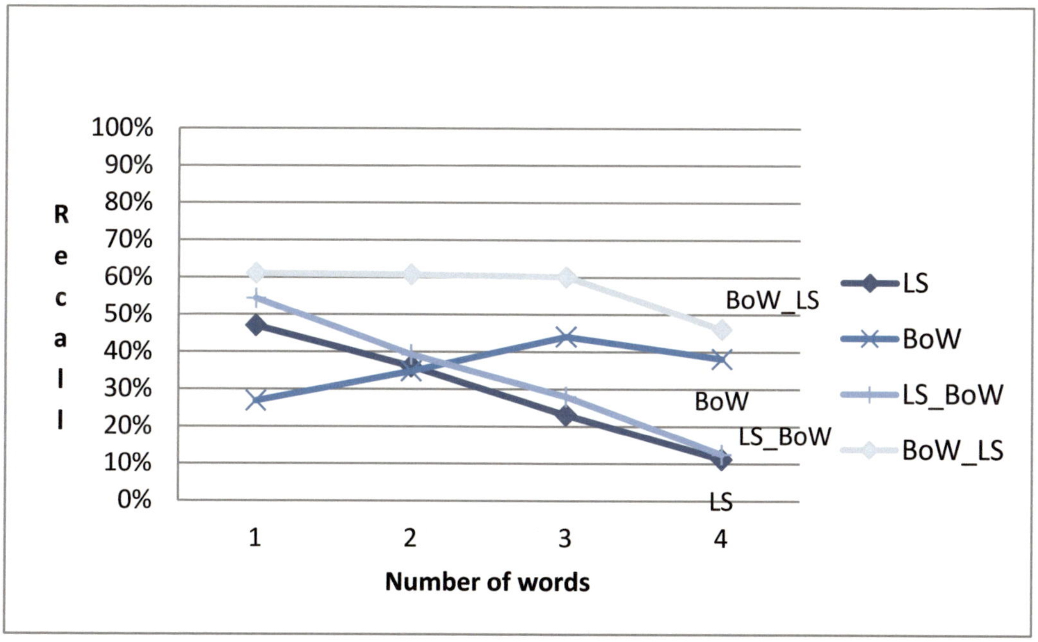

Figure 2. Recall curves according to the size of the query.

The different experiments we performed show that with 38% recall and 42% precision, *Phonemisation* cannot correct all errors : it can only be applied when the query and entry term of the vocabulary have similar pronunciation. However, when there is reversal of characters in the query, it is an error of another type: the sound is not the same and similarity distances such as Levenshtein and Stoilos can be exploited here. Similarly, when using certain characters instead of others ("*ammidale*" instead of "*amygdale*"), string similarity functions are not efficient. The best results (F-measure 64.18%) are obtained with multi-word queries by performing the Bag-of-Words algorithm first and then the spelling-correction based on similarity measures. Due to the relatively small number of correction suggestions (min 1 and max 6), which are manually manageable by a health information seeker, we have chosen to return an alphabetically sorted list rather than ranking them.

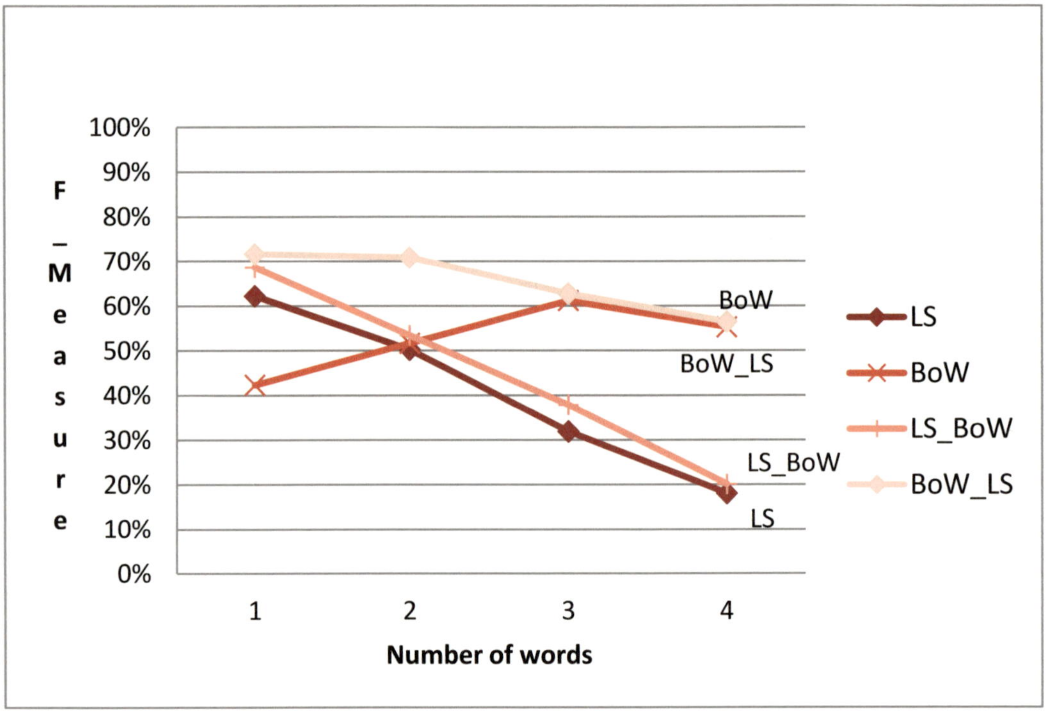

Figure 3. F-Measure curves according to the size of the query.

3.3. Simple heuristics

The complex terms matching is more requiring than simple terms matching. The CISMeF team editorial policy concerning the queries' rewriting consists in maximizing as much as possible the Doc'CISMeF recall. This approach is mainly due to the size of the CISMeF's corpus (n=90,056 *vs.* several million in the MEDLINE database). When all the terms of the query couldn't be recognized as reserved terms or couldn't be corrected by our spell-checker, we have implemented 5 main heuristics:

Step 1. *The reserved terms*: The process consists in recognizing the user query expression. If it matches a reserved term of the terminology, the process stops, and the answer of the query is the union of the resources that are indexed by the term, and the resources that are indexed by the terms it subsumes, directly or indirectly, in all the hierarchies it belongs to. If it doesn't match a reserved term, the query is segmented into seek if it contains one or more reserved terms. The query *'enfant asthme'* is replaced by the Boolean query (*enfant.mr AND asthme.mr*), where *enfant* and *asthme* are reserved terms (*mr*). The reserved terms are matched thanks to the bag of words algorithm independently of the words query order.

Step 2. *The documents' title*: The search is performed over the other fields of the metadata. The title of the documents is considered in priority. The stop words are eliminated and the search is realized over the union of the words of the query with a truncation (*) at the right in the field title (*ti*), as the following: $word_1$*.ti AND $word_2$*.ti for a 2-words query.

Step 3. *Mixing the reserved terms and the titles*: The system seeks if some words are reserved terms or not. A new Boolean query is generated with the fields reserved term (*mr*), if the word is a reserved term, and title (*ti*) if not. The query *'allergie infantile*' is replaced by the Boolean query (*allergie.mr AND infantile.ti*).

Step 4. *Mixing the reserved terms, all fields and adjacency in the titles* : The search is processed over all the fields (*tc*) of the documents' metadata for the words that couldn't be recognized as reserved terms UNION the initial query processed over all the fields with adjacency (*at*) at *n* words with *n=5*(nb words of the query-1)*. The query *'les problems respiratoires des enfants*' is replaced by the Boolean query *[(enfant.mr AND problemes.tc AND respiratoires.tc) OR (problemes respiratoires enfant.at)]*. In this query, the word *enfant* is recognized as a reserved term because it has the same sonority as the reserved term *enfants*. The words *problèmes* and *respiratoires* are searched over all the fields and the initial query *problèmes respiratoires enfants* is searched over all the fields with adjacency of 10 which means that these 3 words shouldn't be distant at more than 10 words.

Step 5. *Mixing the reserved terms, all fields and adjacency in the plain texts* : A plain text search over the documents with adjacency (ap) of n words with n=10*(nb words of the query-1) is realized. The query 'bronchite asthmatiforme' is replaced by the Boolean query (bronchite asthmatiforme.ap) where the words bronchite and asthmatiforme shouldn't be distant at more than 10 words in the plain texts of the documents.

An intuitive scale of interpretation (from Step 1 to Step 5) is available to inform the users about their queries operations and rewritings. By using these simple heuristics, 65% of the queries returned documents (27% by the step 1; 7% by the step 2; 4% by the step 3; 10% by the step 4 and 17% by the step 5).

We describe in the next section how to maximize information retrieval by meta-modeling. The relevance on using multiple medical terminologies to improve information retrieval versus only the MeSH thesaurus is also evaluated.

4. Meta-modeling

To maximize information retrieval through the catalogue, one another enhancement is to gather all the MeSH terms that are related to a given specialty, since they can be dispersed among the 16 MeSH branches. On the other hand, the use of multiple terminologies is recommended [29] to increase the number of the lexical and graphical forms of a biomedical term recognized by a search engine. Since 2007, the CISMeF resources are indexed using the vocabulary of 23 other terminologies and classifications, most of them being bilingual (English and French). To supply health information seekers with the terminologies available in French, these terminologies are accessible through the Health Multiple Terminologies and Ontologies Portal (HeTOP) [31].

4.1. MeSH meta-terms for information retrieval

The MeSH thesaurus is partitioned at its upper level into 16 branches (*e.g.* Anatomy, Diseases). The core of MeSH thesaurus is a hierarchical structure that consists of sets of descriptors. However, these hierarchies do not allow a complete view concerning a specialty. The main headings and subheadings in the CISMeF controlled vocabulary are gathered under meta-terms (*e.g.* cardiology) (Figure 4). Meta-terms (n=73) concern medical specialties and it is possible by browsing to know sets of MeSH main headings and subheadings which are semantically related to the same specialty but dispersed in several trees. Meta-terms have been created to optimize information retrieval in CISMeF and to overcome the relatively restrictive nature of MeSH headings. For example a search on "guidelines" or "virology", where cardiology and virology are descriptors, yield few answers. Introducing cardiology and virology as meta-terms is an efficient strategy to obtain more results because instead of exploding one single MeSH tree, the use of meta-terms results in an automatic expansion of the queries by exploding other related MeSH trees besides the current tree, using the well-known automatic query expansion process. In other words, a query using a meta-term corresponds to the union of all the queries for all the terms semantically linked to it. A comparison of the results of MeSH term-based queries and SC-based queries showed an increased recall with no decrease in precision [33].

4.2. Multiple-terminologies meta-terms

The use of multiple terminologies is recommended [29] to increase the number of the lexical and graphical forms of a biomedical term recognized by a search engine. For this reason, CISMeF evolved recently from a single terminology approach using the MeSH main headings and subheadings to a multiple terminologies paradigm using, in addition to the MeSH thesaurus, vocabularies and classifications that deal with various aspects of health. Among them, the Systematized NOmenclature of MEDicine (SNOMED 3.5), the French CCAM for procedures [34], Orphanet for rare diseases[2] and some classifications from the World Health Organization : the 10th revision of the International Classification of Diseases[3]

---

[2] www.orpha.net

[3] http://www.who.int/classifications/icd/en/

(ICD10), Anatomical Therapeutic Chemical (ATC) Classification for drugs , ICF for handicap, ICPS for patient safety, MedDRA[4] for adverse effects. These terminologies were fully integrated into the CISMeF back-office. They can be used for indexing resources (allowing a more precise indexing) and thus for querying the catalogue. However, the addition of multiple terminologies to CISMeF did not induce modifications in the tasks performed for using, maintaining and updating the catalogue. The richest source of biomedical terminologies, thesauri, classifications is constituted by the Unified Medical Language System (UMLS) Metathesaurus initiated in by the U.S. NLM with the purpose to integrate information from a variety of sources. Nonetheless, the Metathesaurus does not allow interoperability between terminologies since it integrates the various terminologies as they stand without making any connection between the terms in the terminologies other than by linking equivalent terms to a single identifier in the Metathesaurus. The approach in CISMeF has the advantage of combining respect for the original structure of each of the terminologies with a re-grouping of the meta-data inherent in each terminology.

New terminologies have been linked to meta-terms manually by experts in CISMeF: one physician for ICD10, which is partitioned into 22 chapters, and the CCAM; one pharmacist-librarian for ATC, and one medical resident for the terms of the Foundational Model of Anatomy. For instance, the meta-term "*cardiology*" was initially linked to MeSH main headings such as "*cardiology*", "*stents*", and their descendants. With the integration of new terminologies, additional links completed the definition of the meta-term "*cardiology*": links to "*cardiovascular system*", "*Antithrombotic agents*" and others from ATC, links to "*Cardio-myopathy*", "*Heart*" and their descendants from ICD10 and so on.

4.2.1. Test queries

Our aim is to compare the precision and recall of multiple terminologies meta-terms (mt-mt) to MeSH meta-terms (M-mt) in CISMeF. Since mt-mt are based on M-mt plus semantic links to some terms in other terminologies, the query results for M-mt are all included in the query results for mt-mt, which became the gold standard for recall. We have then to evaluate the precision of the query retrieving resources indexed by a term linked to M-mt (MeSH meta-term query), on the one hand, and by a term linked to mt-mt and not to M-mt (Δ query) on the other hand. For this purpose, we build Boolean queries using the meta-terms themselves. For example, for the "*surgery*" meta-term, the MeSH meta-term (M-mt) query is "*surgery[M-mt]*". The Δ query is: "*surgery[mt-mt] NOT surgery[M-mt]*". Retrieved resources returned were assessed for relevance. We detail in the next section the criteria we have used for evaluation.

4.2.2. Evaluations

The resources returned by the CISMeF's search tool using automatic query expansion were assessed for relevance according to a three modality scale used in other standard Information Retrieval test sets: irrelevant (0), partly relevant (1) or fully relevant (2). A physician manually assigned relevance scores (0;1;2) to the top 20 resources returned for

[4] http://www.meddramsso.com

each meta-term query. The results of the evaluation are given in the Table 4. We chose to assign relevance scores to the top twenty resources returned because 95% of the end-users do not go beyond this limit when using a general search engine [35]. For the purpose of assessing meta-terms for Information Retrieval, we have developed a test collection comprising relevance judgments for the top 20 resources returned for a selection of 20 eta-terms queries. Table 4 shows that the queries yielded 118,772 resources, of which 708 were assessed for relevance (0.6%). Weighted precisions for MeSH meta-terms queries and for Δ queries were computed given the level of relevance considered and compared using χ^2 test. Indexing methods and meta-terms were compared too. Relative recall for MeSH meta-terms queries were computed given the level of relevance considered.

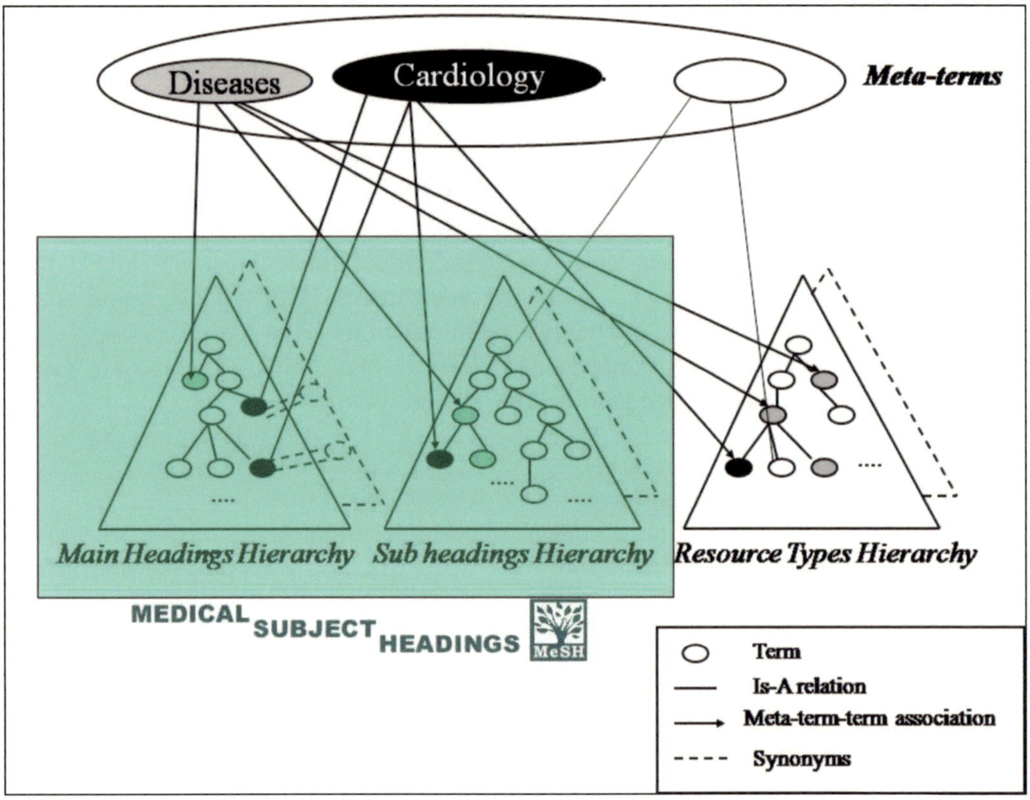

Figure 4. Gathering MeSH *main headings* and *subheadings* under *meta-terms*. *Resource types* are modelled to describe the nature of a resource because of the heterogeneity of resources.

The mean weighted precision of Δ queries was 0.33 and 0.76 for, respectively, full and partial relevance. The mean precision of MeSH meta-terms queries was 0.66 and 0.80 for, respectively, full and partial relevance. The difference between MeSH meta-terms and multiple terminologies meta-terms was significant for full relevance (0.66 *vs* 0.61; $p<10^{-4}$, χ^2) but not for partial relevance (both 0.80; p=0.3, χ^2). The mean recall of MeSH meta-terms queries was 0.92 and 0.86 for, respectively, full and partial relevance. Table 5 shows that, whatever the relevance considered was, results varied significantly according to the indexing method: manual (precision of 0.50 and 0.81 for, respectively, full and partial relevance) perform better than automatic (precision of 0.38 and 0.48 for, respectively, full and partial relevance), and to the studied meta-term.

Meta-Term	Query Type	Nb of documents	Relevance on 20 doc		
			Not	Partially	Totally
Diagnosis	MeSH	13,132	0	2	15
	Delta	350	14	1	5
Toxicology	MeSH	11,980	0	0	20
	Delta	482	16	1	3
Neurology	MeSH	9,325	8	4	8
	Delta	2,168	11	5	4
Infectious Diseases	MeSH	6,557	0	0	20
	Delta	2,573	3	16	1
Paediatrics	MeSH	7,560	4	4	12
	Delta	251	2	4	13
Cardiology	MeSH	5,288	1	0	18
	Delta	2,388	4	10	6
Oncology	MeSH	5,626	0	1	18
	Delta	1,063	2	14	4
Surgery	MeSH	5,504	17	0	3
	Delta	320	5	0	15
Rheumatology	MeSH	4,408	3	8	9
	Delta	856	11	5	4
Gastroenterology	MeSH	4,069	0	0	20
	Delta	1,106	8	11	1
Allergies and Immunology	MeSH	4,598	1	17	2
	Delta	573	2	17	1
Metabolism	MeSH	3,797	14	2	4
	Delta	849	0	2	18
Dermatology	MeSH	3,196	7	0	13
	Delta	1,427	0	4	16
Nutrition	MeSH	3,455	0	1	19
	Delta	1,027	0	9	11
Pneumology	MeSH	3,466	0	7	12
	Delta	584	0	14	6
Gynaecology	MeSH	3,186	6	1	12
	Delta	850	0	1	19
Obstetrics	MeSH	3,063	5	1	12
	Delta	316	20	0	0
Virology	MeSH	3,122	1	11	6
	Delta	257	0	20	0
Total	**MeSH**	**101,332**	**67**	**59**	**223**
	Delta	**17,440**	**98**	**134**	**127**

Figure 5. Relevance of resources retrieved by 18 meta-terms queries on top 20 documents.

Variable	Full Relevance	Partial Relevance
Specific Query (M-mt vs mt-mt)	p < 10-4	p = 0.3
Indexing Method	p = 0.004	$p < 10^{-4}$
Meta-Term	p < 10-4	$p < 10^{-4}$

Figure 6. Determinants of relevance; χ^2 test.

To complete the information retrieval process and to allow interactive query expansion with the health information seeker, we propose in the next section to use "new" knowledge represented as association rules extracted by data-mining process.

5. Knowledge extraction

The knowledge-approach is based upon a data-mining process, called association rules, which can infer "new" relations between medical concepts. A data-mining system may generate several thousands and even several millions frequent association rules, and only some of these will be interesting. In this section we will show how only the most relevant association rules are mined using Formal Concept Analysis and Galois closure. We consider a relevant association rule as being non-redundant with a minimal antecedent and a maximal consequent, which is particularly useful for query expansion.

5.1. Association rules

The discovery of association rules is a widely used technique in data-mining. The general problem was described in [36], in which relations were discovered among pieces of data (called items). An association rule is interesting if it is easily understood by the users, valid for new data, useful, or confirms a hypothesis. The task of association rule mining can be applied to various types of data: any data set containing multiple items.

5.1.1. Definitions

Let I be a set of items, called itemset, and D a database of transactions where each transaction T ($T \in D$) is an itemset. An association rule is an implication rule expressed in the form of: $I_1 \rightarrow I_2$ where I_1 and I_2 are two itemsets $I_1, I_2 \subseteq I$ so that $I_1 \cap I2 = \emptyset$. The rule expresses that whenever a transaction T contains I_1 then T probably also contains $I2$. In other words, the implication rule means that the apparition of the itemset I_1 in a transaction T, implies the apparition of the itemset I_2 in the same transaction. However, the reciprocal implication does not have to happen necessarily. I_1 is called antecedent and I_2 is called consequent.

5.1.2. Support

The support of an association rule represents its utility. This measure corresponds to the proportion of objects which contains at the same time the rule antecedent and consequent. It is possible to calculate the support of an association rule from the support of an itemset. Supp(I_k) the support of the itemset I_k is defined as the probability of finding I_k in a transaction of T:

$$Supp(I_k) = \frac{|\{t \in T / I_k \subseteq t\}|}{|T|} \quad (10)$$

The support of the rule $I_1 \rightarrow I_2$ written as Supp($I_1 \rightarrow I_2$) is calculated as follows:

$$Supp(I_2 \rightarrow I_1) = Supp(I_1 \cup I_2) \quad (11)$$

5.1.3. Confidence

The confidence of an association rule represents its precision. This measure corresponds to the proportion of objects that contains the consequent rule among those containing the antecedent. The confidence of the rule $I_1 \rightarrow I_2$, written as Conf($I_1 \rightarrow I_2$) is calculated as follows:

$$Conf(I_1 \rightarrow I_2) = \frac{Supp(I_1 \cup I_2)}{Supp(I_1)} \quad (12)$$

Two types of rules are distinguished: exact association rules that have a confidence equal to 100%, *i.e.* verified in all the objects of the database and approximate association rules that confidence<100%.

5.2. Data-mining algorithms

Several methods are used to extract all of the association rules from a database. The simplest method consists of enumerating all the itemsets from which all the possible association rules could be generated. The total number of itemsets for a database that contains n Boolean attributes is 2^n. This naïve method is inapplicable to real-life databases. A more efficient method involves computing itemsets that have a support higher than a given threshold. They are called *frequent itemsets*. The association rules extraction time depends on the frequent itemsets extraction time. Several accesses to the database are necessary to compute the number of database objects in which each frequent itemset candidate is contained. The association rules algorithms by level consider in each iteration a set of itemsets of a particular size, *i.e.* a set of itemsets in a level of the itemsets lattice. The following properties are used by these algorithms to limit the number of the itemsets candidates: all of the super-sets of an infrequent itemset are infrequent, and all the subsets of a frequent itemset are frequents [37]. This method is founded on the two-stepped model that finds all of the rules that satisfy user-specified minimum support and confidence: (i) Generate all large itemsets that satisfy minimum support and (ii) From large itemests generate all association rules that satisfy minimum confidence. Apriori algorithm [37] realizes a number of database accesses equal to the size of the larger frequent itemsets. Many researchers have tried to improve various aspects of Apriori, such as the number of passes and accesses to the data-bases or the time efficiency of those passes. We have chosen to adapt the A-Close algorithm [38] in which new bases for association rules are deduced from the closed frequent itemsets and their generators. These bases consist of non-redundant association rules of minimal antecedents and maximal consequents, *i.e.* the most relevant association rules and are defined by using the closure operator of the Galois connection of a finite binary relation. All frequent itemsets and their support, and therefore all association rules, are deduced efficiently from the frequent closed itemsets without accessing the database.

5.3. Extracting knowledge from e-Health documents

Our experiments are carried out on the CISMeF database. An extraction context is a triplet *C= (O, I, R)* where *O* is the set of objects, *I* is the set of all the items and *R* is a binary relation between *O* and *I*. Applying this model to our database, the objects are the indexed e-health documents. Each document has a unique identifier and a set of associated descriptors. These descriptors may be MeSH main headings and associations between MeSH main headings and MeSH subheadings. The relation *R* represents the indexing relation between an object and an item, *i.e.* a descriptor that belongs to *I*. We studied different extraction contexts by applying and adapting the A-Close algorithm such as the context of categorized documents, according to the user type and to meta-terms. There is an average of 6.5 descriptors by document in CISMeF with a minimum of 1 and a maximum of 300. This constraint on the number of descriptors *i.e.* the size of the set of items has been considered in the implementation phase of the A-Close algorithm. Indeed, A-Close works on databases with a maximum of 12 items. We have added another requirement to the implementation to avoid long time generation: maximal size of the closed itemsets is fixed to 300 items as it corresponds to the maximum number of descriptors for the documents. As an output, the association rules may be visualized in a file or automatically added to the database to be used in the information retrieval process, mainly by interactive query expansion.

5.3.1. Extracting knowledge from all the database

- *Case 1*: In the first case, let *I* be the set of main headings (MH), which, via *R*, are used to index a subset *O* of 11,373 documents. The 11,373 documents were selected at random. We have fixed the support threshold as minsup=20 and the confidence threshold as minconf=70%. A total of 11,819 rules were mined (2,438 exact with confidence=100%; 9,381 approximate with confidence≥70%). The number of rules is too high to be manually analyzed by our experts (physicians or medical librarians).
- *Case 2*: In the second case, let I be the set of main headings (MH) and subheadings (SH) associated with the set of documents O. $I=\{MH\}\cup\{SH\}$. We obtained 16,976 rules (5,241 exact; 11,738 approximate). The same conclusions are drowned from the case 1 : too numerous rules to be evaluated manually.

- *Case 3*: In the third case, *I* is the set of the associations of main headings and subheadings (MH/SH) related to the documents. *I={[MH/SH]}*. Association rules between couples of (MH/SH) are more precise than association rules between main headings, and between main headings and subheadings since a subheading specifies a particular aspect of a main heading. With the same thresholds as in cases 1 and 2, the number of rules is 2,565 (648 exact rules; 1,917 approximate rules).

The extracted association rules in the precedent cases are related to the medical domain. To obtain more precise rules we performed experiments on categorized documents according to groups of users: students in medicine, health professionals, and general public to evaluate the influence of categorization on the generation of association rules.

5.4. Categorizing documents according to health information seekers

In CISMeF, mainly three types of health information seekers are categorized: professionals, students in medicine, patients and lay people. We consider three major resource types: guidelines*, education* and patients*. We also consider two kinds of itemsets: the set of major main headings I={MH*} and the set of major (main heading/subheading) pairs I={[MH/SH]*)}. The collection is detailed in Table 6.

Resource type	Documents	Items	Min	Max	Mean
Guidelines*	2,727	MH*	1	64	5.21
		MH/SH*	1	70	6.12
Patients*	3,272	MH*	0	25	1.63
		MH/SH*	0	30	1.82
Education*	3,610	MH*	0	25	2.22
		MH/SH*	0	34	2.73

Table 4. Description of the collections of documents.

For all contexts, the minimum support threshold was fixed to minsup=20 and the minimum confidence threshold was fixed to minconf=70% (Table 7). We obtained association rules between major main headings MH* in the first context where I={MH*} and between [MH/SH]* pairs for I={[MH/SH]*}. For the major resource types patients* and education* all association rules (100%) are between two MHs* and between [MH/SH]* i.e. one descriptor in the antecedent and one descriptor in the consequent. For the major resource type guidelines*, 24% of the rules are between more than two descriptors. The characteristics of documents may explain these results: average descriptors were from 1.63 to 2.22 for patients* and education* whereas they were from 5.21 to 6.12 for guidelines*.

Resource types	Item=MH*				Item=[MH/SH]*			
	Nb rules	ER	AR	Nb pairs	Nb rules	ER	AR	Nb pairs
Guidelines*	50	12 24%	38 76%	38 76%	39	8 20.51%	31 79.49%	35 76%
Patients*	20	9 45%	11 55%	20 100%	19	8 42.1%	11 57.9%	19 100%
Education*	23	6 26.09%	17 73.91%	23 100%	25	13 52%	12 48%	25 100%

Table 5. Number of rules, exact rules (ER), approximate rules (AR), and number of pairs.

5.4.1. *Evaluation of the extracted knowledge*

Not all of the association rules extracted were evaluated: according to the context extraction and the itemset I there are more or less association rules. The more the collection is specialized, and the itemset size is reduced, the less we have association rules to evaluate. As defined, an interesting association rule confirms or states a new hypothesis [38].

Here, we proposed to combine background domain knowledge with simple statistical measures used traditionally in association rules mining for evaluation. We considered several cases of interesting association rules according to relations between MeSH headings. As these relations are defined between two main headings and between two subheadings, we considered only the association rules between two elements. Hence, an interesting existing association rule could associate: a (in)direct son and its father (relation FS); two descriptors that belong to the same hierarchy (same (in)direct father) (relation BR); two descriptors with See Also relation (relation SA). These rules are automatically classified thanks to the MeSH structure. The other rules that satisfy the minsup and minconf are then considered as «new» interesting association rules.

Exact association rules, except for collection patients*, are mostly new interesting rules: from 62.5% to 87.4%. Therefore, existing rules are mainly from the patients* collection: 77.8% for MH* and 75% for MH/SH*. However, approximate rules, are mostly existing rules (Table 8). Subjective interest measures are based on expert knowledge about the data, *i.e.* that of physicians and medical librarians in this context. New interesting rules for the contexts MH* and [MH/SH]* pairs are evaluated manually. 93.8% (resp. 84.8%) of the interesting new rules with conf=1 (resp. conf≥0.7) between major descriptors are validated.

Resource types	Items	Exact rules				Approximate rules			
		Existing knowledge			New	Existing knowledge			New
		FS	BR	SA		FS	BR	SA	
Guidelines*	MH*	-	-	4 33.3%	8 66.7%	2 5.3%	7 18.4%	10 26.3%	12 31.6%
	MH/SH*	1 12.5%	1 12.5%	1 12.5%	5 62.5%	3 9.7%	3 9.7%	9 29%	13 42%
Patients*	MH*	-	5 55.6%	2 22.2%	2 22.2%	2 18.2%	2 18.2%	4 36.3%	3 27.3%
	MH/SH*	-	5 62.5%	1 12.5%	2 25%	2 18.2%	2 18.2%	3 27.3%	7 36.3%
Education*	MH*	1 16.7%	1 16.7%	-	4 66.6%	2 11.8%	6 35.3%	3 17.6%	6 35.3%
	MH/SH*	1 7.7%	-	1 7.7%	11 87.4%	2 16.8%	3 25%	2 16.8%	5 41.4%

Table 6. Association rules evaluation according to the MeSH structure

5.5. Knowledge-based query expansion

Our objective is to re-use the numerous association rules that we extracted from the CISMeF database into the information-retrieval process by query expansion. We use Interactive Query Expansion. For example, the association rule *breast cancer* → *mammography* is extracted from the corpus because the keywords *breast cancer* and *mammography* are frequently used together to index the documents. This association rule is as a "new" one because it doesn't exist in the domain knowledge which is, in our case, the MeSH thesaurus. When applying the association rule *breast cancer* → *mammography* on a query containing the term *breast cancer*, an interactive query expansion proposes to the user e-health documents related to *mammography* to complete the search. In medicine and health-related information, [40] have already investigated an efficient algorithm for association rule mining using the MeSH thesaurus. They adopted a MeSH-indexed representation of MEDLINE records, but the evaluation of the interest of the mined associations with respect to the task of PubMed retrieval improvement was not considered by the authors. In [41] many other works on information retrieval and query expansion in the biomedical domain are also presented. Methods to perform query expansion with promising results involve mining user logs [41] and constructing user profiles. And another study on logs in PubMed for searching biomedical and life-science literature online has been performed by [43].

In the literature, a number of methods for performing query expansion have been developed. The solutions given are based mainly on two approaches. The first is the augmentation of query terms to improve the retrieval process without user intervention. The second is the suggestion of new terms to the user which can to be added to the original query to guide the search towards a more specific document space. The first case is called automatic query expansion whereas the second case is called semi-automatic query-expansion. In [44], the authors tried to evaluate and compare the efficiency of the two methods. Despite the fact that their experiments were based on simulations and not on real human users in most of the cases, the results of the experiments showed that the interactive query expansion method gave more control to the searcher who knows her utility better than any automated system. Researchers also turned to methods such as lexical co-occurrence [45]. Lexical co-occurrence is the process of developing relationships between words based upon their co-occurrence in documents. The similarity of the method we have proposed here with lexical co-occurrence is that the source, which provides the candidate terms for expansion, is the set of the retrieved documents as opposed to some knowledge structure as in thesaurus-based approaches. As a consequence, if the user chooses terms that do not yield results from the expected domain, the terms suggested by the query-expansion algorithm are unlikely to be helpful to the user. A solution may be a simple spell-checker.

5.6. Evaluating query expansion based on association rules

Many ways of navigation and information retrieval are possible in the catalogue. The most used is the simple search (free text interface). As stated in the section 2, it is based on the subsumption relationships. A query (a word or an expression) can be matched with an existing concept. In this case, the result of the query is the union of the resources that are indexed by the concept, and the resources that are indexed by the concepts it subsumes, directly or indirectly, in all of the hierarchies it belongs to. The co-occurrence tools developed for information retrieval bring the terms which frequently appear in the same documents closer together. These terms thus have a semantic proximity. This technique was used very early to allow query expansion. By analogy, association rules may be exploited in a search engine by carrying out an interactive query expansion. This helps the user to formulate his query by using the result of a query to reformulate, filter and re-orientate the query by exploiting the terms related to his query terms. In fact, the user can select suggested terms sets to add them to his initial query. It is useful in the case of non-precise information needs. IQE requires user implication. We developed a web-based evaluation tool of the IQE used by a set of 500 users which are subscribers of the weekly letter "What's new" of CISMeF. 20 queries, and for each one a set of medical terms derived from the extracted association rules were proposed. The evaluation was performed thanks to a Likert scale. The results (76% of the users were satisfied by the propositions) demonstrate the usefulness of this approach. An expanded query by association rules contains more related terms. By using the vectorial model, for example, more documents will be located and this treatment increases recall. In addition, association rules are indication on the possible definition of a term or its context.

6. Conclusions

We have presented in this chapter useful methods to help health information seekers to find resources on the Internet which is the most popular way used nowadays. The experiences were carried out on the CISMeF catalogue in French, but are reproducible for other e-health applications in other languages. These methods include simple ones such as heuristics and spell-checking, and more sophisticated ones such as knowledge extraction from e-health documents.

Author details

Lina F. Soualmia, Badisse Dahamna and Stéfan J. Darmoni
CISMeF & TIBS-LITIS EA 4108, Rouen University &Hospital, France

7. References

[1] Hou J, Zhang Y. Effectively finding relevant web pages from linkage information. IEEE Transactional Knowledge Data Engineering 2003; 15(4), 940–951.
[2] Liu, B. Web data mining: exploring hyperlinks, contents and usage data. Springer. 2007
[3] Keselman A, Browne AC, Kaufman DR. Consumer health information seeking as hypothesis testing. Journal of American Medical Informatics Association 2008; 51(4):484–495.
[4] Koch T. Quality-controlled subject gateways: definitions, typologies, empirical overview. Online Information Review 2000; 24(1):24–34.
[5] Abad Garcia F. A comparative study of six European databases of medically-oriented web resources. Journal of the Medical Library Association 2005; 93(4):467–479.
[6] Douyère M, Soualmia LF, Rogozan A, Dahamna B, Leroy JP, Thirion B, Darmoni SJ. Enhancing the MeSH thesaurus to retrieve French online health resources in a quality-controlled gateway. Health Information Libraries Journal 2004; 21(4):253–261.
[7] Baker T. A grammar of Dublin Core. D-Lib Magazine 2000; 6(10).
[8] Nelson SJ, Johnson WD, Humphreys BL. Relationships in Medical Subject Heading. In: Relationships in the Organization of Knowledge, 2001, eds. Kluwer Academic Publishers, pp. 171–184.
[9] Soualmia LF, Darmoni SJ. Combining Different Standards and Different Approaches for Health Information Retrieval in a Quality-controlled Gateway. International Journal of Medical Informatics 2005; N°74; vol (2-4); pp. 141–150.
[10] McCray AT, Ide NC, Loane RR, Tse T. Strategies for supporting consumer health information seeking. Proceedings of the 11th World Congress on Health Informatics, Medinfo 2004; pp.1152–1156.

[11] Grannis SJ, Overhag MJ, Mc Donald C: Real world performance of approximate string comparators for use in patient matching. Studies in Health Technology and Informatics 2004; 107:43–47.

[12] Levenshtein V. Binary codes capable of correcting deletions, insertions and reversals. Soviet Physics Dokl 1966; 10:707–710.

[13] Yarkoni T, Balota D, Yap M. Moving beyond Coltheart's N: a new measure of orthographic similarity. Psychonomic Bulletin & Review 2008; 15(5):971–979.

[14] Soualmia LF. Towards intelligent information retrieval with query expansion knowledge-based methods. PhD thesis 2004; INSA Rouen.

[15] Hodge VJ, Austin J. A comparison of a novel neural spell checker and standard spell checking algorithms. Pattern Recognition 2002, 11(35):2571–2580.

[16] Damereau FJ. A technique for computer detection and correction of spelling errors. In Communication of the ACM 1964; 7(3):171–177.

[17] Peterson LJ. A note on undetected typing errors. Communications of ACM 1986. 29(7):633–637.

[18] Kuckich K. Techniques for automatically correcting words in text. ACM Comput Surv 1992, 24(4):377-439.

[19] Kernigham M et al. A spelling correction program based on noisy channel model. In proceedings of conference on COmputational LINGuistics, 1990. vol. 2.

[20] Brill E, Moore RC. An improved error model for noisy channel spelling correction. In proceedings of the Association for Comput. Linguistics 2000; 286–293.

[21] Toutanova K, Moore RC. Pronunciation Modeling for Improved Spelling Correction. In proceedings of the Association for Comput. Linguistics 2002; 141–151.

[22] Boyer C, Baujard V, Griesser V, Scherrer JR. HONselect: a multilingual and intelligent search tool integrating heterogeneous web resources. International Journal of Medical Informatics 2001, 64(2–3):253–258.

[23] Crowell J, Long Ngo QNG, Lacroix E. A frequency-based technique to improve the spelling suggestion rank in medical queries. Journal of the American Medical Informatics Association 2004, 11(3):179–185.

[24] Peters L, Kapunsik-Uner JE, Nguyen T, Bodenreider O. An approximate matching method for clinical drug name. AMIA Annual Symposium 2011, in press.

[25] Wilbur JW, Kim W, Xie N. Spelling correction in the PubMed search engine. Information retrieval 2006. 9:543–564.

[26] Stoilos G, Stamou G, Kollias S. A string metric for ontology alignment. In Proceedings of the International Semantic Web Conference, 2005; 624–637.

[27] Yujian L, Bo L. A normalized Levenshtein distance metric. IEEE Transactions on Pattern Analysis and Machine Intelligence 2007, 29(6):1091–1095.

[28] Winkler W. The state record linkage and current research problems. Technical report: Statistics of Income Division, Internal Revenue Service Publication 1999.

[29] Moalla Z, Soualmia LF, Prieur-Gaston E, Lecroq T & Darmoni SJ. Spell-checking queries by combining Levenshtein and Stoilos distances. Proceedings of Network Tools and Applications in Biology 2011, online.

[30] Wagner MM. An Automatic Indexing Method for Medical Documents. Symposium on Computer Application in Medical Care. 1991:1011–1017.

[31] Grosjean J, Merabti T, Dahamna B, Kergourlay I, Thirion B, Soualmia LF & Darmoni SJ. Health Multi-Terminology Portal: a semantics added-value for patient safety. Studies in Health Technology and Informatics 2011, 166:129-138.

[32] Soualmia LF, Griffon N, Grosjean J & Darmoni SJ. Improving Information Retrieval by Meta-modelling Medical Terminologies. Proceedings of 13th Conference on Artificial Intelligence in MEdicine 2011, 6747:215–219.

[33] Gehanno JF, Thirion B, Darmoni SJ. Evaluation of Meta-Concepts for Information Retrieval in a Quality-Controlled Health Gateway. In: Proceedings of the American Medical Informatics Association symposium 2007; pp. 269–273.

[34] Trombert-Paviot B, Rodrigues JM, Rogers JE, Baud R, van der Haring E, Rassinoux AM, Abrial V, Clavel L, Idir H. GALEN: a Third Generation Terminology Tool to Support a Multipurpose National Coding System for Surgical Procedures. In International Journal of Medical Informatics 2000; 58-59: 71–85.

[35] Spink A, Wolfram D, Jansen BJ & Saracevic T. Searching the web: the public and their queries. Journal of the American Society Information Science Technology 2002, 52(3):226–234.

[36] Agrawal R, Imielinski T & Swami AN. Mining association rules between sets of items in large databases. In Proceedings of the ACM SIGMOD International Conference on Management of Data 2003; 207–216.

[37] Agrawal R. & Srikant R. Fast algorithms for mining association rules in large databases. In Proceedings of the VLDB Conference 1994; pp. 478–499.

[38] Pasquier N, Taouil R, Bastide Y, Stumme G & Lakhal L. Generating a condensed representation of association rules. Journal of Intelligent Information Systems 2005, 24(1):29–60.

[39] Fayyad UM, Piatetsky-Shapiro GP, Smyth P & Uthurusamy R. Advances in Knowledge Discovery and Data Mining 1996. American Association of Artificial Intelligence.

[40] Kahng J, Liao WHK & McLeod D. Mining generalized term associations: count propagation algorithm. In Proceedings of the KDD workshop 1997, pp.203–206.

[41] Prince V & Roche M. Information Retrieval in Biomedicine: Natural Language Processing for Knowledge Integration 2009. IGI Global.

[42] Cui H, Wen JR & Ma WY. Query expansion and classification by mining user logs. Knowledge and Data Engineering 2003, 15 (4):829–839.

[43] Lu Z. & Wilbur WJ. Improving Accuracy for identifying related PubMed queries by an integrated approach. Journal of Biomedical Informatics 2009; 42:831–838.

[44] Ruthven I. Reexamining the potential effectiveness of interactive query expansion. In Proceedings of the 26th Annual International ACM SIGIR Conference on Research and Development in Information Retrieval 2003; pp. 213–220.
[45] Vechtomova O, Robertson S. & Jones S. Query expansion with long-span collocates. Information Retrieval 2003, 6(2), 251–273.

Chapter 4

Codified Knowledge and Decisions in a Major eHealth Project: Efforts to Introduce the Electronic Health Record in Quebec

Duncan Sanderson, Marie-Pierre Gagnon and Julie Duplantie

Additional information is available at the end of the chapter

http://dx.doi.org/10.5772/50322

1. Introduction

Electronic health records (EHR) are being implemented in countries around the world, as the hope is that they will allow health personnel to have more timely access to information about patients and their medical history, and to improve quality of care. These objectives have translated into major expenditures and effort in order to try to implement national EHRs. The United States, for example, passed the Health Information Technology for Economic and Clinical Health (HITECH) provisions of the American Recovery and Reinvestment Act of 2009 [1]. In England, from 2003 to 2010, the government spent $20.6 billion on the National Programme for Information Technology (NPfIT) [2]. In Canada, it has been reported that $1.6 billion has been alloted to this effort [3].

Along with expenditures and efforts to implement these systems, there has recently been an interest in the evaluation of national projects to implement an EHR, both in terms of the results that have been achieved and the road that has been taken [2-4]. Although evaluations of the implementation of national EHRs are still relatively scarce, there have been some remarkable efforts. For example, in the case of England, Greenhalgh et al. [2] note that the national EHR project was expensive and well behind its implementation schedule, and indicate that its success was limited. Furthermore, these authors point out that "policymakers appeared to overlook many of their recommendations and persisted with some of the NPfIT's most criticized components and implementation methods" [2](p. 533). To explain the limited uptake of their recommendations, they note that policymakers generally failed to learn from the evaluations that had been commissioned.

For their part, Stroetmann et al. [4] identify good practices and lessons learned in European countries, while noting that progress has not been simple: "... implementing them (eHealth strategies) has proven to be much more complex and time-consuming than initially anticipated. In addition, the complexity of eHealth as a management challenge has also been vastly underestimated" [4](p.1349).

In Canada, a similar broad assessment effort has also occurred recently [3]. A short explanation of certain aspects of the Canadian health system, as they relate to the EHR, could be useful at this point. Canada is a federation of provinces and territories, which are primarily responsible for providing health services to the citizens living in their geographic territory. The individual health organizations (private clinics, public hospitals) have a main role in maintaining the patient's record, although each provincial Ministry of Health has oversight over the public hospitals and, to a lesser extent, some influence on private physician's practices. The provincial and federal Ministries of Health set policy and decide if they want to support EHR projects. However, at the turn of the century (2001), the federal government wanted to insure that patient record systems would be compatible so that a citizen who moved from one province to another could still provide a record of treatment to his or her new physician. This resulted in an organization (Infoway) and a large federal fund to facilitate the development of interoperable systems. This initiative will be further described in a particular section below.

If we return now to the recent analysis of this federal initiative (Infoway), Rozenblum et al. [3] observe that "Canada continues to lag behind other Western countries in adopting electronic health records" [3]. These authors report that, across the provinces and for 2009, only 36% of physicians were using an EHR, and that this was much lower than for countries such as Australia, the United Kingdom, New Zealand, and the Netherlands. The authors carried out a set of telephone interviews of key informants from three provinces across Canada (not including Quebec), and these informants indicated a number of reasons for the poor rate of implementation: lack of an e-health policy (federally and in concert with the provinces), inadequate involvement of clinicians, failure to establish a business case for using electronic health records, a focus on national rather than regional interoperability, and inflexibility in approach.

In this chapter we wish to take a different approach, by examining decisions that have been made during the process of implementing a provincial EHR and the influence that codified knowledge may have had on those decisions. Our general goal is to document, and if possible, gain deeper understanding of the reasons for which scientific evidence in particular may be considered or not in EHR projects. We will argue that in Quebec, but probably not unique to it, key decisions regarding EHR implementation have not always been based on available knowledge, and this could help to explain the limited success of EHR projects here and perhaps elsewhere.

Currently, under the label of evidence-based medicine, there is substantial interest in, and effort by, health researchers to examine empirical evidence in order to identify actions and conditions that are most likely to result in positive outcomes for patients. This chapter builds on this strategy. Where possible, we will point out certain research results, expertise, and evaluation conclusions (which we will call the codified knowledge) that were available to decision-makers at the time of their decisions. We will identify specific occasions during which the available knowledge influenced decision-makers (or was available and did not have an influence), and we will explore the reasons for which this may or may not have occurred.

2. Methodology

Our presentation and analysis centre on decisions, projects, and events, along with aspects of the political, technological, and social context in Quebec, Canada. As we have indicated earlier, because of provincial jurisdiction in the area of health in Canada, significant decisions were made in this area by the provincial government, and for this reason, the province is a useful unit of analysis. The Federal government also funded some projects, and these too represented significant decisions. These are the main decisions that will be considered here, although we also recognize that many other decisions took place and likely affected the projects, such as the choice of partners, the creation and composition of steering committees, the project objectives, the technology used, as well as implementation, training, and recruitment strategies.

The analysis is based on a multiple case study approach [5] which examined the evolution of representative EHR projects in the Province of Quebec from the first large scale pilot project at the beginning of the 1990's until just before the development of the current Quebec EHR project in the late 2000s (le Dossier santé du Québec, or DSQ). Although this approach limits the amount of detail that we can provide for any one project or event, we believe that this longer historical view is also useful. Because of the scope of the current project (the DSQ) and ongoing analysis of it (for example, annual reports by the Auditor General of Quebec), we will not include it here, except for an early initiative that was part of it. Further analysis may eventually find that many of our conclusions also apply to it.

For the analysis here and because of space limitations, a subset of projects or actions were chosen for this chapter which are either representative of similar projects or which, retrospectively, can be considered to have been a significant event (see Table 1). The choice of projects and activities that are discussed here was reached by consensus among the authors. The projects selected also allow us to present and discuss several factors which influenced the uptake of codified knowledge by the EHR projects in Quebec.

By codified knowledge, we mean knowledge that has been written down in the form of reports or articles. The particular type that we are mostly concerned with here is scientific evidence that has been produced by evaluation studies of projects, or research into the actual benefits of an EHR, or factors that affect the implementation of EHR projects. Other pertinent codified knowledge may have been produced in fields other than scientific research. In the case of the EHR, an important area of knowledge consists of an understanding of legislation that controls the storage or transmission of a patient's clinical information. Rather than to stretch the notion of scientific evidence in order to accommodate this type of knowledge, we prefer the more general expression of codified knowledge.

For each case study, we analyzed public descriptions, evaluations, and reports concerning the set of projects and events. This information was supplemented by semi-structured interviews with decision-makers, which allowed us to explore the context in which decisions were made, how available knowledge was actually used (or not) to make decisions, and factors which influenced its use. A total of 31 interviews were completed with key decision-makers who were selected because of their involvement in EHR projects either as policy-makers, evaluators, or project leaders. For the first case study, one of the authors (JPF) co-directed the evaluation of it. In relation to the final case study, two of the authors (MPG and JD) observed several meetings between December 2007 and March 2009 and conducted informal interviews with members of a consulting team.

For each project or activity discussed, we will briefly note its objectives, the major decisions that were made, whether certain forces may have influenced the decisions, the types of difficulties the project or activity may have experienced, and the knowledge that was gained from it. The following table identifies the projects and activities that will be presented.

Project/Activity	Approximate Time Period
The Rimouski Smart Health Card Project	1993-1995
The Role of the *Commision d'accès à l'information* (CAI)	1993 -
Canada Health Infostructure Partnerships Program	2001-2003
Changes in the Provincial Laws	2001, 2005
Canada Health Infoway (inclusion of Quebec)	2004 -
The *RSVP*: a change management strategy	2007-2009

Table 1. Major Projects and Activities in Quebec, on the Road to an EHR

3. Presentation of the case studies

3.1. The Rimouski smart health card project

One of the earliest electronic health record projects in Quebec took place in a small city in Quebec, Rimouski, from 1993 to 1995. This was one of the first large-scale experiments of this type in the world, although it built on a similar concept that was active in France at the time (for a later description of a similar concept, see [6]). The Quebec government decided to encourage the project, provided financial assistance to it (4 million dollars Canadian), and also sponsored an evaluation [7]. The RAMQ (the provincial organization which manages health insurance, pays private physicians for their interventions, and issues health cards) was the main project manager and associated several stakeholders such as professional associations. Proponents of the project hoped that it would help to meet the objectives of the dominant ideology of the time, which was a shift to ambulatory care (see, for example [8]), and the creation of a better continuum of services by the set of professionals that a patient could see. A report from an important consultation on the reform of health care in Quebec (known as the *Commission Rochon* [9]) had also recommended that a trial be carried out with the card. Two implicit sub-objectives of the experiment were to decrease drug interactions, and to decrease the duplication of lab tests.

A group of academic experts was set up in order to plan the implementation of the pilot smart health card project. They consulted the literature (which was scarce at the time), along with a research group that had implemented the technology in France [10]. The group in Quebec included a variety of researchers from various fields (health services, political science, evaluation, information technology), as well as medical experts. Significant consideration was given to clinical processes and inter-professional collaboration. A local physician was also involved in the project team as a strategy in order to increase the acceptance by the medical community. The project team used knowledge gained from European projects in particular, to inform the implementation of this pilot project. The project was envisioned to be a way to produce new knowledge about the benefits of the smart card for the health care system, but also to help develop strategies that would be useful for a future large scale implementation.

A specific health card was used for this project, and had a smart chip on it that could record information. The concept was essentially to create a portable personal medical record. For example, patients' allergies or reactions to medication could be noted on the card. Citizens who wanted to participate had to apply and consent to the project (this consent could be withdrawn later), and an office was created to facilitate this. Health professionals needed a personal identification number (PIN) in order to access information on the card, as well as a card reader and IBM microcomputer. It is useful to remember that, at the time, pharmacists often had experience using a computer, but this was not the case for physicians or nurses. When a patient went to visit a health professional, they could present the card and so the information on the card could be shown to him or her, and if suitably equipped and inclined, the professional could in turn add to it. As well, a computer application was offered to pharmacists so that they could check for potential drug interactions. At the end of the project, there were 7248 users (a portion of the city's population), along with 299 physicians, pharmacists, and nurses (almost all of the health professionals who had been identified as potential users) [7].

Overall, 73% of the population who had a card used it. Among these patients, about half used it with a pharmacist and a physician [7]. One of the decision aids that was most used (often by pharmacists) was an application that checked for potential drug interactions. The rate of use increased until July 1994, and then decreased, and this coincided with a decision to not buy more smart cards for the project. As well, there were indications that the use of two different computer systems was an irritant, that use of the card increased the time needed for a consultation, and there were occasional problems updating information on the card. In the summer of 1995, a sample of patients and health professionals were polled, and they generally indicated that the card facilitated the communication of health information, in a secure manner. In spite of the problem related to the need to update information, more than half of the health professionals felt that it provided quicker access to information, allowed them to provide better recommendations, and were satisfied with its quality. As well, many indicated that certain characteristics of the project, in particular the slowness of the system, did not facilitate its systematic use.

Some of the professionals felt that the smart health card provided benefits that out-weighed the irritants and disadvantages, whereas for others, the advantages were not sufficient. Most found it relatively easy to use, although the system was found to be too slow. In general, the physicians and pharmacists indicated that the system contributed to a decrease in drug interactions [7].

The evaluation report included a number of recommendations. For example, such a system needed to be compatible with a computer system in a physician's office or a pharmacy, so as to minimize work for the professional. As noted previously, the information provided by a system should also be up-to-date, and consideration should be given to ways to encourage patients to adopt the behavior that project planners hoped they would have, such as presenting the card (this affected whether the information was indeed up-to-date). Local support for the users was also indicated to be a critical factor, as well as the implication of a local leader. As well, the confidentiality of the health information had to be insured.

In a later analysis of the project, Aubert and Bernard [11] add that the training requirements of the health professionals was a significant aspect of the project. As well, they note that physicians' offices were generally not equipped with computers. In addition, according to these authors, reflection about changes in clinical practices that could maximize the use of such technology seemed to be absent (although it was clear that the project hoped to decrease drug interactions, and reduce the number of lab exams).

Although the evaluation included the identification of actions which could contribute to the generalization of the project elsewhere, there was no such immediate follow-up. A later project in the health region of Laval (north of Montreal), from 1999 to 2001, used another smart card, although patient health information was stored in a database managed by the RAMQ. The Quebec government considered the smart card to be a viable approach, and continued to consider its potential use as late as 2002. In particular, the RAMQ announced in 2001 that within three years it would provide the card to 80% of the population [11].

3.2. The role of the Commision d'Accès à l'Information (CAI)

In Quebec, the CAI (Commission of Access to Information; our translation) was created in 1982, and had a significant influence on events and practices in relation to the EHR. In this section we will describe this organization and some of its activities in relation to electronic health records, and briefly comment on its influence in relation to the development of the EHR in Quebec. From the outset, we should note that this organization was not associated with a single electronic patient record project, but rather several of them. As well, the information it produced was not scientific evidence in the sense that we are generally using it here, but could be considered to have produced pertinent codified knowledge. As we hope to show, the organization produced information of a particular kind, but nevertheless, information that project proponents and the provincial government had to consider.

In 1982, a law was passed in Quebec, which had an objective of instituting better management and protection of information concerning individuals, which was held by the government. An organization was created at the same time to administer this law (the CAI) and it was "responsible for overseeing compliance with the obligations imposed upon public bodies concerning the collection, storage, use and communication of personal information" (http://www.cai.gouv.qc.ca/index-en.html). Health and social service institutions, which created databases that contained health information, fell under the mandate of this organization. Furthermore, the CAI was authorized to comment on draft bills in this area and to assess pilot projects.

Because of this mandate, the CAI decided to analyze various EHR pilot projects that took place in Quebec from 1990 to approximately 2005, as well as on proposed provincial legislation. To be clear, it was a decision-maker in this way, since it opted to comment on the EHR projects and hoped to steer them in a way that would allow them to be compliant with various laws, but it did not have a direct role in the selection of projects which were carried out. As an example of one activity, it wrote a report on the Smart Card and its trial in Rimouski [11]. Although the CAI considered the approaches taken in this project to be useful, problems with the implementation of the card were also noted, such as allowing nurses and pharmacists to share a card, and the fact that it consisted of a partial patient record.

A later, more general study carried out by the CAI in 2001 summarizes their examination of several pilot projects and outlines their general concern: "The transfer of clinical information and the right to privacy are not contradictory. However, their conciliation is complex and fragile, especially when they are implemented" [12](our translation, p. 2). A particular concern was also presented in this report, in that the authors indicate that the provincial health insurance organization, the RAMQ, should not be the organization that handles a centralized health record, and it discussed the reasons that motivated it to take this position.

This 2001 report also summarized the state of legislation in this area: "In relation to the laws that relate to the protection of personal health information, these are numerous, haphazard, sometimes contradictory, and often insufficient in relation to these new health technologies" [12](p. 35). An analysis of the state of the current legislation (in 2001) was also carried out. At the end of this analysis, several questions were raised about the legislative foundation for certain practices concerning the communication of information, such as who would be responsible for the information that is collected, and the regulations that would control this. The obvious call for further legislation which was contained in this report eventually lead to some proposed laws, and to subsequent analysis by the CAI of these proposed laws.

In general, one could conclude that the work of the CAI had an influence on the legislation that framed the creation of the current provincial EHR project. For example, in 2004, a law was proposed that would have modified the main law in Quebec that governs health and social services, and the CAI provided an analysis of this [13]. One of the recommendations in it was that staff in a health organization should not be able to provide patient information to staff in other health organizations without the consent of the patient. As well, the authors recommended that the provincial health insurance organization (RAMQ) should not create a database that would document the medications used by citizens.

The fact that the CAI examined several projects and proposed laws over an extended period of time indicates that senior managers in the CAI decided that this was an area that needed to be examined and monitored. It was also clear that this organization was sufficiently independent from the elected government in order to critically examine the activities of the government. Since many managers of pilot projects informed the CAI of their projects and actively solicited its opinion about a project, this suggests that these project managers were concerned that their projects could potentially contravene existing legislation. At the time, managers felt that the rules were ambiguous about what a project needed to do in order to conform to existing legislation, and many meeting hours were spent discussing what to do about this problem.

3.3. Canada Health Infostructure Partnerships Program

At the turn of the millennium (2000-2002), the *Canada Health Infostructure Partnerships Program* (CHIPP) was a two-year, $80 million, 50-50 shared-cost program with an objective of supporting collaboration, innovation, and renewal in health care delivery through the use of information and communication technologies. One of the specific areas that was funded was the creation of EHRs. Project applicants were required to complete a literature review, and to include an evaluation.

In Quebec, three EHR projects were funded through the CHIPP program. One of these, called MOXXI, or the Medical Office of the XXI century, was a research project to examine the potential benefits of an electronic prescription and drug management system for primary care physicians [14]. Two of the project objectives were to streamline the prescription process and to improve patient safety. Another aspect examined was the time requirements and other ergonomic issues related to the use of the system. One of the interesting questions implicit in this project was whether such a computerized system would be a help or a hindrance for the physician. This sort of question had generally not been asked before, and is still very rare in Canada. As one of the outcomes of the project, the authors concluded [15]: "However, there are considerable barriers to developing the interfaces necessary with community-based pharmacies to permit exchange of information between physicians and pharmacists" [15].

A second CHIPP project called RIGIC was essentially a project to create a networked EHR system which would be shared between two hospitals, for oncology patients. One of the outcomes of the project was that shared protocols (between the hospitals) had to be established in terms of access and confidentiality procedures. New policies and procedures also had to be developed in relation to this, including the development of a consent management system. As well, the participants became more aware of the importance of change management, and the need for recurrent funding in order to transition the research project into an ongoing operation.

A third project, the SI-RIL project, consisted of the development of an integrated network system in a health region (the health region of Laval, north of Montreal), for ambulatory patients. This system was designed to enable the sharing of physician orders and patient health information among health workers in the region, with a view to regional co-ordination of care. The participants were: the local hospital, four community health centres (CLSCs), and more than one hundred general physicians.

During the course of the project, a number of factors were observed which influenced its development [16]. For example, the Minister of Health changed repeatedly during this period, and it was stated that these changes increased the level of uncertainty. As well, health professionals were not necessarily available to participate in the project, so consulting them was not an easy matter.

One of the outcomes was a set of standardized clinical forms which were agreed to by health professionals, such as a form to assess patient autonomy. Another was that project proponents realized that it was difficult to comply completely with certain outdated laws, and they communicated this problem to provincial authorities. Still another outcome was that participants noted that significant resources were required in order to manage the change process. Observations were gathered about impacts on the work processes, and a recommendation was made to the effect that these had to be considered. Quite a few documents were produced by the project, which can be taken to be an indicator of a high amount of consultation, discussion, and analysis which took place during the project.

It would appear that the SI-RIL project was one of the most advanced primary care EHR projects in Canada at the time. All other networked EHR projects in Quebec involved a small group of hospitals (there were a couple of networked hospital projects at the time). An evaluation of part of the SI-RIL project was also carried out by a research group [17]. For example, the authors highlighted the fact that these were very complex projects, and that any one of three types of problems (technological, organizational, clinical) could lead to the end of the project [17]. In addition, also noted in the report, was the desire of project participants to find a way to avoid illegal transmission or storage of patient information.

In the case of the RIGIC and SI-RIL projects, the regional health authority was closely integrated in the project planning and execution. We mention this since the regional health authority has regular communication with the provincial Ministry of Health. This highlights the fact that the provincial government was fully informed of the difficulties met by the proponents of the three projects, along with the outcomes, at least by 2002, when the project funding ended.

Another significant dimension of these projects was that all of them were based on networked health information systems. Patient information was being made available to professionals in different organizations, without patient intervention. This fact contrasts with a concomitant provincial plan to develop an electronic patient card.

3.4. Changes in the provincial laws

In December 2001, the provincial government proposed a law that would have created a provincial smart card and replaced the existing health card. It should be pointed out that the Laval region had also been involved in a second electronic health card project, which began in 1999, and this project was again sponsored by the RAMQ [12]. For those who proposed the law, this project provided an example of the type of technology that would be used. One of the technological differences with the Rimouski project was that a patient's clinical information was centralized in a databank managed by the RAMQ.

The purpose of the proposed law was to allow the development of a provincial electronic patient record, enabled by the patient's use of a smart card, although the patient record would have only been a summary. A law was also necessary in order to allow easier communication of health information between health organizations, which were subject to restrictions because of laws that were active at the time. With the proposed law, the RAMQ would have become the government's manager of the smart card, and the card would have included both administrative information (the name, address, and date of birth of the patient), and health information. In contrast with the Rimouski project, this information was to be centralized in a database. As part of the legislation development process, the government included a public consultation on the law.

More than 50 groups and individuals responded with written comments about the proposed law [18]. There was a public debate about the law in the media, which gave rise to what one commentator considered to be a sterile debate often based on misconceptions [18]. Professional organizations, such as the provincial Nurses Association, Association of Pharmacists, and an association of physicians, also joined this debate. One of the specific criticisms of the physicians was that a centralized database should not be created, and that a government organization should not manage health summaries (a comment directed at the RAMQ) [19]. The CAI also questioned the inclusion of administrative and clinical information together in one database, and the management of this database by the RAMQ. They also reminded the government of the ongoing need (implicitly beyond this law), to widen the legislation that would frame the management and access to health information. It highlighted the recent creation of family medicine groups, and suggested that such groups could be the focus of efforts to computerize health information, since most health services were provided by primary care services. Finally, it issued a clear warning about the project:

> ... the law that the government has tabled entails solutions that could jeopardize the confidentiality of health information. The text has a number of grey zones which do not allow us to know with precision the orientations that will be followed. [20] (p. 28, our translation)

In one of our interviews, a government official had this to say about the public debate at the time:

> We could say that the proposed law was a major error, the law that was tabled became the object of several controversies; several philosophers, the citizens thought that we wanted to create a 'big brother', that it was a way for the RAMQ to gain power over the health system; the physicians did not want to be controlled and were concerned about the way it was developing. (government official)

The result of the controversy and the questions that were raised was that the government withdrew the proposed legislation. In theory, it could have revised the proposed law, but perhaps because of the extent and range of the opposition, it decided to abandon it completely.

Two and a half years later, and under a new government, another law was proposed in December 2004 (proposed law number 83). Although the CAI and other organizations again tabled reports about the proposed law, there was relatively little public opposition to it, and it was adopted almost a year later. It was clear, however, that it had taken many years for the government to respond to the request from the CAI to enact such a law. With this law, clinical information would now be managed by regional health organizations (there are 18 health regions in Quebec), and this regional organization, even though it was part of the government, was separate from the RAMQ.

3.5. Canada Health Infoway

In 2001, Canada Health Infoway (Infoway), was created in order to accelerate the adoption of compatible electronic health records across the country. This organization was funded by the federal government, but accountable also to the provincial and territories' health ministers, all of whom were represented on a Board of Directors. Projects in the provinces were generally funded equally by Infoway and provincial governments. Over ten years, $1.6 billion Canadian was allocated to this project [3].

One of the main priorities of Infoway was to incite provinces to adopt technologies which would allow patient records in one province to be available to health providers in other provinces. Another rationale was that it would be possible to save money and time by having common technologies deployed across provinces.

In a report provided in 2005, consultants to Infoway proposed a three-phase approach to health technologies. The first phase would consolidate patient data for viewing by health professionals, the second phase would allow the documentation of care and provide basic decision support, and the third phase would allow physician orders and decision support. The estimated cost at that time of reaching the 3rd phase was $10 billion.

In was not until 2004 that the Quebec government decided to join Infoway. Informants indicated that Quebec did not participate in Infoway from 2001 to 2004, and at the end of this period, the situation was such that it was the only province which had not yet joined the project. One senior official indicated that the discussions during this period were "very, very political." The decision to join Infoway was made in 2004, and was taken by a newly elected Liberal provincial government (the previous ruling party was the Parti Québécois, a sovereignist party). This decision implied that Quebec would need to harmonize its EHR plans with those of Infoway and have its projects and deliverables approved by Infoway in order to receive the funding contribution by the federal government. In particular, local companies which had been supplying technology to Quebec health institutions, would have to be compliant with the standards defined by Infoway (for an analysis of the development of standards in Canada, see [21]).

One of the influences that seemed to affect the Quebec government's decision to join Infoway, seemed to be the possibility of obtaining financial advantages. As previously noted, the federal government provided a significant grant to Quebec (and other provinces) as a financial incentive. A form of group purchase of certain technologies also became possible. As a government official commented: "In the end, Quebec chose the same solution

(PACS technology) which saved us about 16 million, because they (the technology company) gave us a discount".

3.6. The *RSVP*: An evidence-based change management strategy

In the subsequent years, work continued with the planning and development of a province-wide EHR, and culminated in the launch of another pilot project in Quebec City, in May 2008. In this pilot project, a patient record system was used that was to be expanded across the province, the DSQ or Dossier santé du Québec. The DSQ had been developed within the Infoway framework, thus the federal government funded about half of it.

From 2007 to 2009, the DSQ project proponents carried out an implementation strategy, which was called the Network for Peer Support, or *RSVP* (*Réseau de soutien et de validation par les pairs*). The RSVP strategy aimed to facilitate the appropriation of the DSQ throughout the province through the mobilization of an interdisciplinary group of healthcare professionals (general practitioners (GPs), specialists, nurses and pharmacists). These groups were represented by clinical champions for each of the 18 health regions of the province. Although the pilot project was only taking place in Quebec City, the belief behind the RSVP activity was that the project would soon be extended to the rest of the province, and so it was necessary to include professionals from all the regions. The selection of these champions was made by the various regional health agencies according to a set of criteria, including their credibility, recognition within their peer group, and their interest in informatics. The stated roles of the RSVP members [22] were to:

1. Participate in the elaboration and the realization of the change management strategy at the provincial level, by validating and adapting the promotion tools developed by the DSQ team to the needs and expectations of the professional groups that they represented;
2. Promote the appropriation of the DSQ within their provincial professional association;
3. Identify the challenges and obstacles to DSQ implementation in their region and help to identify solutions;
4. Exchange information with other RSVP participants regarding the DSQ in their region, provide tips for facilitating appropriation by their peers.
5. Ensure constant communication with their peers regarding the DSQ and answer their questions;
6. Work in collaboration with other RSVP members, the regional DSQ group, and other local groups in order to find solutions to challenges and difficulties identified by the DSQ change management team or their peers;
7. Make recommendations and participate in decisions which concern all aspects of the appropriation of the DSQ in their region.

In the DSQ change management documentation [23], it was clear that this strategy was directly informed by evidence in the literature related to the importance of change management and consideration of the critical role that clinical leaders play in the implementation of large scale EHR projects. As well, the managers of the RSVP had requested and received presentations by Quebec experts on change management. The DSQ team had contracted a consulting group, and this group proposed the RSVP strategy. For example, RSVP members were offered training and support in order to prepare a promotion plan for the DSQ in their region. RSVP members were also invited to answer a questionnaire, which measured various aspects pertinent to change management.

Over the course of the RSVP strategy, the need for an interdisciplinary team was expressed but once this team was created, new challenges arose. The rationale for an interdisciplinary team was never directly expressed in the written internal documents, but interviews with the change management team indicated that this decision was based mainly on the perception that resistance from nurses and pharmacists could become an important obstacle, if the promotion of the DSQ was left solely to physicians.

However, important limits to the interdisciplinary team started to appear after a first large group meeting. The physicians who had already had extensive discussions about the project, had a more extensive understanding of the project, compared to the nurses and pharmacists who were new to the group. The large number of participants at the interdisciplinary meetings (more than 50 RSVP members plus the DSQ management group and invited speakers) made it much more formal than the earlier meetings which had only included physicians. RSVP members from the three professional groups agreed that it was extremely difficult to have constructive exchanges within such a large group. They also believed that issues specific to each profession (remuneration for physicians, access to diagnostic data for pharmacists, or responsibility for data entry for nurses) could not be easily addressed in an interdisciplinary group. A solution that was put in place was to alternate meetings specific for nurses, pharmacists, and physicians, and the interdisciplinary meeting. This strategy was costly given the fact that the DSQ team had to reimburse participants' travel and time. A teleconference was then used, given these constraints, but many RSVP members found that the exchange did not progress as well as with the in-person meetings.

This project was one of the first to formally include a team of experts in change management, and to develop an explicit change strategy. Still, the impact expected from the RSVP did not occur. This was mainly due to factors unrelated to the implementation strategy, such as the delays in the DSQ technology. In fact, the pilot project had revealed several problems, notably the slowness of the system. Therefore, the plan of deploying other pilot projects in other regions had to be altered during the course of the RSVP. Participants were kept informed about the global DSQ strategy but, according to our interviews, it became very difficult for them to know exactly what was going on at the provincial level, and to play their role of DSQ representative within their region. According to one physician, it was "impossible to know who was holding the steering wheel and to know where we were going".

The RSVP was an exemplar of a provincial government strategy informed by best practices in change management and the implementation of innovations. However, it took place in an environment that was extremely complex and was based on a technology that was not mature. The change from a group composed mainly of physicians to an interdisciplinary group led to a profound change in the social dynamics, which also hampered the realization of the RSVP's mission.

4. Discussion of the case studies

An analysis of the projects and events described above will now be carried out with a view to highlighting the possible influence of codified knowledge in relation to decisions that determined the projects and events described above. The main decisions that we have highlighted are the ones in which a government or government organization (example, Health Canada) decided to fund a particular project, or to propose or withdraw a proposed law. In the case of the CAI, several decisions were made to examine and to comment on the patient information practices of various projects.

However, when presenting several of the various case studies, it also became apparent that a host of actors were also making various other decisions that affected the projects. Various actors, both individuals and organizations, had to decide whether to become active partners, what steps would be taken to insure the confidentiality of patient information, what technologies would be used and which companies would be hired, whether they would resist or support a project, how potential participants would be addressed so as to encourage their participation, and so on. Many decisions were made in relation to which codified knowledge could have played a role or not. At this point we can only indicate that we are cognizant of all these other decisions that were taking place, and which collectively also determined the outcome of any given project.

Decisions concerning which projects to fund were most likely being made by senior government officials or, perhaps in some cases, elected representatives who were in cabinet (the cabinet is formed by the government ministers). Elected government officials would certainly have been involved in the decision to propose or withdraw a given law. At the project definition phase, however, key decisions would have been made by other decision-makers. For example, the Rimouski project required a coalition of local physicians, local health officials, private companies, along with support from the RAMQ and certain officials within the Ministry of Health. The contributions to the project description (and the decision of these actors to participate in it) would have been influenced by the knowledge, beliefs, and interests of these participants. On the other hand, the decision to fund the project was likely taken by the Council of Ministers. In this regard, we should note that we did not have direct access to either of these groups at the time when decisions were being made (with the exception of the RSVP project). This could be an area for further historical research (i.e., what information did senior officials provide to the Minister of Health for the projects and activities discussed here). Still, a certain number of general observations can be made about the possible influence of codified knowledge on certain decisions that were taken.

In general, a series of real-life, in-situ pilot projects were an integral part of the 16-year period we are analyzing here (1993-2009). These projects allowed the provincial government to develop extensive experience with the challenges and issues associated with EHR projects. The projects were not part of a coordinated plan, but were rather local initiatives which were financed by the provincial (in the case of the Rimouski project), or primarily federal government (CHIPP projects), or both (DSQ project). Although the primary goal of these projects was not to develop "original knowledge", the goal was certainly to create large-scale, real-life tests of technology in an actual clinical context. The hope was that if the project was a success, that it would continue and the technology would become integrated into daily use. If it was not a success, it was implicit that participants would learn from the experience. Some thought had been given to how to maximize learning or knowledge development, since an evaluation was a part of most if not all of the projects.

One general observation that can be drawn from the various experiments is that project promoters seemed to believe that the technological systems that had been developed were ready for real-world experimentation. Smaller scale tests to simulate the real-world demands on the systems seemed to be either absent, or inadequate. This could have been learned with the Rimouski project. In some of the projects, the project proponents appeared to think that the technology would "sell itself", and be relatively easy to implement, although the importance of attending to the users' reactions to technology and to change management did not seem to have been assimilated until the time of the RSVP project. This can be inferred especially from the CHIPP project reports about the "lessons learned". Project promoters seemed to be surprised that medical personnel would require computer systems that responded quickly to requests for information, that users would need extensive training and technical support, and that there could be mixed reactions to the technology on the part of patients, citizens, and personnel.

These sorts of warnings were not new, even in the 1990s, and we would argue that these issues were common knowledge at the time in fields as diverse as management of information systems (for example [24]), computer supported cooperative work [25], and the design and implementation of IT [26]. Our interviews indicated that not all project promoters consulted with experts from these fields, and this was an obvious shortcoming. For their part, we found little evidence of senior government officials or decision-makers having consulted with those who had implemented IT systems in hospitals. Although the systems in place in hospitals at the time may have been simpler than the ones developed for the projects described here, lessons from the implementation of hospital systems could probably also have been applied in these projects.

In the case of the Rimouski project, little scientific evidence about the benefits of EHR or electronic health card projects existed in the early 1990s. So, other than knowledge that was available in other fields or from experiments such as the one in France, it was clear that project planners had relatively little scientific evidence from health researchers that could have been used to orient the implementation strategy. Indeed, $4 million dollars was spent on an innovation that did not have a track record in the health field. Very little information was available concerning the clinical impact of the innovation. It is useful to remember that, at this time, the few scientific articles on the subject generally reported on individual hospital systems [27, 28], or announced the advent of medical computerization and its benefits [29, 30]. For example, the latter write in the summary of their article: "The electronic medical record in the ambulatory setting will be a force to be reckoned with during the 1990s. The increased quality of the medical record will lead to an increased quality of patient care at a fairly level cost (no long-term increase)." Still, the state of the literature at the time did not provide solid support for the hope, on the part of project proponents and government decision-makers, that an EHR system could be readily introduced into a whole city, or would lead to clinical improvements. One of the purposes of the project was precisely to create better knowledge about the feasibility and the requirements for such a system. Even today, although several countries have managed to attain a high level of use of an EHR by clinicians, there is still debate about its clinical impact [31].

Although the evaluation report about the Rimouski project included analysis of use by health personnel, and analysis of perceptions about the usefulness of the information that was made available through the system, it did not analyze clinical changes that could have been used to assess this project or to inform later ones. On the other hand, and in contrast with later projects, a significant number of dissertations were produced in relation to the project. The authors of the evaluation report also identified factors that would likely affect any further projects to introduce the smart card on a wider scale.

Another surprising event was that the concept and technology that was active in the Laval electronic health card project became the basis for the law that was proposed in late 2001. According to one account, even more that a year after the project began (in May, 2001), only 290 patients out of the 1678 who had received a card, actually used it [12]. In spite of results which were not favourable, and in spite of clear concerns on the part of the CAI with respect to the Laval project [12], the provincial cabinet decided to propose legislation which used this project as a model for a province-wide system. The low rate of adoption by patients could be considered to be empirical evidence that should have lead officials and cabinet to question the concept on which the proposed legislation was based. A similar viewpoint was expressed publicly in a newspaper article that appeared in the newspaper *Le Devoir*, May 7th 2001, well before the legislation was tabled: "The trial of the electronic health card [in Laval], which Quebec wants to extend to the whole province, was not a clear success."

As well, the simultaneous experimentation with a different network technology in the RIGIC project and two other simultaneous projects to create a patient record shared between hospitals, which we have not discussed here, obviously did not alter the government's plans at the time. One of these was called Arc-en-ciel, and was a project financed by the Quebec Ministry of Health, in order to create an EHR shared by three hospitals. Thus the Ministry of Health must have been aware that certain projects were experimenting with another type of EHR technology, and that knowledge about this type of technology was in the process of being developed. For whatever reason, perhaps because of concerns about the cost of this technology, it decided that it was not worthwhile to wait for the results of these projects.

In 2001, the Quebec government decided to not participate in Infoway, then later, after the change in government in 2004, to participate. The rationale provided by informants for the two decisions suggested that these were not influenced by scientific evidence. The first decision, to not participate, seemed to stem from a desire to not accept the terms and requirements stated by the federal government. The second one, to participate, appeared to be motivated primarily by financial considerations: the opportunity to acquire additional funding for an EHR in Quebec, and to a lesser extent, to obtain better deals from vendors through group purchases. The question of whether or not an EHR could contribute to positive clinical results did not appear to be discussed in either case. The participation of Quebec in Infoway provided opportunities to obtain information about the strategies and progress made elsewhere, required that Quebec document and demonstrate the achievement of intermediate objectives for external observers, and some knowledge transfer may have been an unintended consequence of participation in it.

With the RSVP project, senior government officials demonstrated an understanding of the importance of developing and executing strategies that would facilitate the implementation of an EHR. They had clearly come into contact with and had expended effort to better understand scientific literature on change management and the management of the implementation of technology. The spheres of considered knowledge had expanded to include new strategies for communicating with, consultation of, and preparation of primary actors. The problem that arose was that the communication activities that were undertaken appeared to be premature.

The actors who participated directly in a given project undoubtedly gained practical experience, but it is difficult at this point to evaluate the extent to which expertise developed by individuals in one project may have been exploited in subsequent projects. Still, our impression is that the level of re-employment of personnel was low since new project groups were formed for each of the EHR projects. This is also consistent with the findings of a study that examined information sharing between health informatics projects in Quebec and noted that there was little knowledge exchange between the projects [32].

Other mechanisms for learning or transfer of knowledge and expertise could have been formal and informal meetings. Again, we are not able to determine the extent to which people who were involved in one project may have had contact with those who were planning subsequent projects. It is worthwhile noting though, that a series of annual conferences were held in Quebec on the theme of computer systems and healthcare, and several presentations were made about the projects discussed here. This conference was a forum for the exchange of information. The Quebec Society of Biomedical and Health Informatics (SoQIBS) was created in 2001 and is still organizing annual meetings on topics related to health information technologies (see http://soqibs.org/). This initiative is supported by researchers, clinicians, commercial enterprise, and government.

5. Strengths and limitations

This multiple case study is one of the first studies to examine the development and implementation of an EHR in a jurisdiction over an extended period of time. Although it does not constitute a full historical analysis, which is still needed, it adds to the knowledge base concerning factors that have contributed to the limited success of large-scale EHR implementations [2-4]. We used information from multiple sources, including scientific and technical literature, evaluation reports, policy documents, analysis of proposed laws, newspaper articles, and semi-structured interviews with stakeholders involved in the projects.

We are also keenly aware that we have not been able to fully document the myriad decisions and influences that culminated in a decision to fund any particular project. Someone who wishes to do this would be advised to concentrate initially on a single project. Also, although we have suggested that codified knowledge seemed to have relatively little influence in most projects, one means of partially verifying this would be to obtain initial project descriptions and to check to see what scientific evidence may have been cited in order to justify project objectives and orientations (we did not have such documents). What we suspect is that other forms of "evidence" may have sometimes been used (for example, what people were told by project promoters during short visits to sites which may have had less than a fully implemented EHR, or impressions of how an EHR may change care processes).

The selection of the cases under study was made by consensus among the authors, based on criteria such as the relative novelty of the project or activity and its importance in relation to later developments. However, the study of other EHR cases could potentially bring new insights [2]. Our analysis may also have been limited by the fact that some projects took place up to twenty years ago. We relied on documents that were published, as well as on the recall of individuals who participated in the projects. Thus, our analysis could be limited by the available documents and/or recall bias from interviewees. The presentation of several case studies has necessarily limited the amount of detail that could be provided for any one of these. However, the consideration of an extended period of time, triangulation of information, and the validation of our interpretation of each case with several respondents who represented different perspectives (policy-makers, researchers, and project leaders) likely helped us to gain a richer understanding.

6. Conclusion

This chapter examined decisions that have been made during the process of implementing particular EHR projects in the Province of Quebec, Canada. As we have indicated, a significant number of projects took place over the sixteen years that we have considered here, and these involved a variety of locations, objectives, and technologies.

Perhaps the most surprising characteristic of this period is the limited impact of codified knowledge on projects and activities, and this seems to be a problem that has been experienced in other countries as well [2]. Technological shortcomings and the need to insure that the user has a positive experience, both noted in the evaluation of the Rimouski project, cropped up again in later projects. Observations were repeated from one project to another about the need to invest in change management. Warnings from the CAI about the need to update legislation and to consider the complexity and depth of concerns about approaches to safeguarding health information did not seem to be fully considered. Pertinent knowledge developed outside of the health field was not transferred into it. Large scale pilot projects helped to develop codified knowledge but this was not fully exploited over time. However, a note of caution is required here, as these conclusions are tentative, and further investigation and analysis is required.

In the last two decades, there has been a strong emphasis within the health field concerning, on the one hand, the importance of basing decisions and medical practice on scientific evidence, and on the other, the importance of effective knowledge transfer. Unfortunately, in Quebec and elsewhere, it has also taken two decades for these two philosophies and practices to gradually permeate into the multiple and interconnected dynamics that may eventually produce a provincial and a Canadian EHR.

Author details

Duncan Sanderson
Research Centre of the Centre hospitalier universitaire de Québec, Québec, Canada

Marie-Pierre Gagnon
Research Centre of the Centre hospitalier universitaire de Québec, Québec, Canada
Faculty of Nursing, Université Laval, Québec, Canada

Julie Duplantie
Department of Social and Preventive Medicine, Faculty of Medicine, Université Laval, Québec, Canada

Acknowledgement

The initial study on which part of this chapter is based was funded by the Canadian Institutes of Health Research (grant # 200603MOP-159757-KTE-CFBA-111141). This study was approved by the institutional review board of the Centre hospitalier universitaire de Québec (#5-06-09-02). We would like to acknowledge the contribution of Dr. Jean-Paul Fortin who provided thoughtful comments on this chapter, and Dr. France Légaré and Dr. Michel Labrecque who made useful suggestions concerning the study on which this chapter is based. We would like to sincerely thank all the people who participated in the interviews.

7. References

[1] Blumenthal D, Tavenner M. (2010) The "meaningful use" regulation for electronic health records. N Engl J Med. 363(6):501-4.

[2] Greenhalgh T, Russell J, Ashcroft RE, Parsons W. (2011) Why national eHealth programs need dead philosophers: Wittgensteinian reflections on policymakers' reluctance to learn from history. Milbank Q. 89(4):533-63.

[3] Rozenblum R, Jang Y, Zimlichman E, Salzberg C, Tamblyn M, Buckeridge D, et al. (2011) A qualitative study of Canada's experience with the implementation of electronic health information technology. CMAJ. 183(5):E281-8.

[4] Stroetmann KA, Artmann J, Stroetmann V. (2011) Developing national eHealth infrastructures--results and lessons from Europe. AMIA Annu Symp Proc. 2011:1347-54.

[5] Stake RE. (1995)The Art of Case Study Research. Thousand Oaks: Sage Publication.

[6] Morris S, Cooper J, Bomba D, Brankovic L, Miller M, Pacheco F. (1995) Australian healthcare: a smart card for a clever country. Int J Biomed Comput. 40(2):101-5.

[7] Fortin JP, Joubert P, Morisset J, Kirouac S, Bérubé J, Papillon MJ, et al. (1996)Évaluation du projet québécois d'expérimentation de la carte santé à microprocesseur : rapport final.: Régie de l'assurance maladie du Québec. Available: http://www.fmed.ulaval.ca/dmsp/fileadmin/fichiers/MEDECINE_SOCIALE_ET_PREVENTIVE/Personnel_enseignant/Professeurs_reguliers/Fortin_Jean-Paul/Rapport_final_complet_-_RAMQ.pdf Accessed June 2012.

[8] Bonneville L. La mise en place du virage ambulatoire informatisé comme solution à la crise de productivité du système sociosanitaire au Québec (1975-2000). Ph. D. thesis. Montreal: Université du Québec à Montréal.; 2003.

[9] Commission d'enquête sur les services de santé et les services sociaux. (1988) Rapport de la commission d'enquête sur les services de santé et les services sociaux. Les Publications du Québec.

[10] Beuscart R, Dufresne E, Grave C, Haye MP. (1994) Carte à micro-processeur et Informatique Médicale.

[11] Aubert B, Bernard JG. (2002) Les cartes à puce dans le domaine de la santé : leçons et défis. Gestion. 27(3):81-7. Available: http://www.jgbernard.com/files/rg_aubert_bernard_les_cartes_a_puce_dans_le_domaine_de_la_sante_2002.pdf. Accessed April 12.

[12] CAI (Commission d'accès à l'information). (2001) Évaluation du projet vitrine carte santé de Laval de la régie de l'assurance maladie du Québec (RAMQ). Available: http://www.cai.gouv.qc.ca/documents/CAI_REEV_vitrine_carte_sante_RAMQ.pdf. Accessed April 2012.

[13] CAI (Commission d'accès à l'information). (2005) Mémoire sur le Projet de loi no 83. Available: http://www.cai.gouv.qc.ca/documents/CAI_M_PL-83.pdf. Accessed April 2012.

[14] Bartlett G, Tamblyn R, Huang A, Kawasumi Y, Petrella L, Dufour E. (2003) Evaluation of standardized tasks for primary care physicians using the MOXXI electronic prescribing and integrated drug management system. AMIA Annu Symp Proc.786.

[15] MOXXI (2005) Project MOXXI. Available: http://www.hc-sc.gc.ca/hcs-sss/pubs/chipp-ppics/2004-moxxi/synopsis/index-eng.php. Accessed April 2012.

[16] SI-RIL. (2005) Project vitrine PRSA. Available: http://www.hc-sc.gc.ca/hcs-sss/pubs/chipp-ppics/2004-prsa/index-eng.php#som. Accessed April 2012.

[17] Sicotte C, Moreault, M.P., Farand, L. (2004) Technologies de l'information et soins médicaux de première ligne. Report R04-05. Available: http://www.irspum.umontreal.ca/rapportpdf/R04-05.pdf. Accessed April 2012.

[18] Péladeau P. (2002) Avant-projet de loi sur la carte santé du Québec - La démocratie aux prises avec le gouvernement électronique. Le Devoir, 6 aout 2002. Available: http://www.ledevoir.com/non-classe/6599/avant-projet-de-loi-sur-la-carte-sante-du-quebec-la-democratie-aux-prises-avec-le-gouvernement-electronique. Accessed April 2012.

[19] Association médicale du Québec. (2002) Mémoire de l'Association médicale du Québec à la Commission des affaires sociales sur l'avant projet de loi sur la carte santé. Available: http://www.amq.ca/fra/pdffiles/AMQcarteSante.pdf. Accessed April 2012.

[20] CAI (Commission d'accès à l'information). (2002) Mémoire concernant l'avant-projet de loi sur la carte santé au Québec. Available: http://www.cai.gouv.qc.ca/08_avis_de_la_cai/01_pdf/memsante.pdf. Accessed April 2012.

[21] Kuo M-H, Kushniruk A, Borycki E. (2011) A Comparison of National Health Data Interoperability Approaches in Taiwan, Denmark and Canada. ElectronicHealthcare. 10(2):e14-e25.

[22] Bureau du Dossier de santé du Québec. (2008) Dossier de santé.com vol 2(no 1): www.dossierdesante.gouv.qc.ca.

[23] Bureau du Dossier de santé du Québec. (2008) Dossier de santé.com. Vol 2(no 4): www.dossierdesante.gouv.qc.ca/filearchive/84b1012d6cf7e3715e607b1f57fbbc1b.pdf.

[24] Cooper RB, Zmud RW. (1990) Information technology implementation research: a technological diffusion approach. Management Science 36(2):123-39.

[25] Grudin J. (1988) Why CSCW applications fail: problems in the design and evaluationof organizational interfaces. Proceedings of the 1988 ACM conference on Computer-supported cooperative work; Portland, Oregon, United States. 62273: ACM; p. 85-93.

[26] Ehn P. (1989) Work Oriented Design of Computer Artifacts. Hillsdale, NJ: Lawrence Erlbaum.

[27] Bleich HL, Beckley RF, Horowitz GL, Jackson JD, Moody ES, Franklin C, et al. (1985) Clinical computing in a teaching hospital. N Engl J Med. 312(12):756-64.

[28] Burke JP, Classen DC, Pestotnik SL, Evans RS, Stevens LE. (1991) The HELP system and its application to infection control. J Hosp Infect. 18 Suppl A:424-31.

[29] Benson DS, Reimlinger G. (1991) Electronic medical records in the ambulatory setting: the quality edge. J Ambul Care Manage. 14(1):78-87.

[30] McDonald CJ. (1988) Computer-stored medical record systems. MD Comput. 5(5):4-5.

[31] Holroyd-Leduc JM, Lorenzetti D, Straus SE, Sykes L, Quan H. (2011) The impact of the electronic medical record on structure, process, and outcomes within primary care: a systematic review of the evidence. J Am Med Inform Assoc.

[32] Fortin J-P, Grant A, Lavoie G, Reinharz D, Douillard D, Messikh D, et al. (2003) Éléments pour un plan d'informatisation du réseau de la santé. Rapport sur les enseignements de projets de recherche et d'expérimentation d'envergure.

Chapter 5

Ontological Architecture for Management of Telemonitoring System and Alerts Detection

Amine Ahmed Benyahia, Amir Hajjam, Vincent Hilaire and Mohamed Hajjam

Additional information is available at the end of the chapter

http://dx.doi.org/10.5772/3158

1. Introduction

Telemonitoring (health monitoring, Home Health Care) is a branch of telemedicine that aims to restore independent living in their homes, to people suffering from various diseases and disabilities that would force them to a hospitalization or placement in specialized institutions (patients suffering from certain chronic diseases, disabilities, but also the frail elderly) [1].

This emerging area has led to much research during the past two decades and led to some development of systems that allow the maintenance to their homes of these people. To prevent the risks associated with lack of medical support "presential", technological systems must be implemented to provide graduated responses, adapted to individual cases, but it must in addition ensure respect of privacy of the person and not disrupt their lifestyle.

These systems must be open, able to integrate various technologies, at the same time flexible enough to adapt to the case of each patient, and to reflect changes in health state of a person.

Telemonitoring is based on the transmission and interpretation of medical indicators (clinical, radiological or biological) collected by the patient himself or by a health professional (doctor, nurse, etc) [2]. They can be interpreted by a health professional, or through programs and specialized software. The interpretation may lead to the decision to intervene with the patient or just provide advices.

Among the benefits of telemonitoring: The friendliness of the technology. A better understanding of the health status and better control of symptoms that give a sense of security. Economic system by minimizing hospitalizations and unnecessary displacement.

Telemonitoring is characterized by the use of vital data sensors necessary for diagnosis as blood pressure, weight, temperature, blood oxygen saturation, etc. These sensors are, in most cases, wireless (Bluetooth, Wi-Fi, etc) for more freedom of movement and portability [3]. Other sensors can be used as behavioral sensors (for example if the patient's spirit to climb stairs that affects blood pressure), or environmental sensors such as ambient temperature.

The smart house system can easily take advantage of existing technologies in home automation to facilitate the completion of certain tasks by the person, for example, unlock a door in an emergency, turn on or turn off lights, adjust the heating. Moreover, robots can help the person to perform certain daily tasks. Thus, a manipulator arm can be mounted on a wheelchair or on a mobile robot, to press a button, a lever handle door or catching. Also, depending on conditions, the system should take into account the therapeutic machines: syringe pump, infusion, dialysis machine or pill. It should be noted that these machines load their own sensors and can also participate in the task of data acquisition.

In earlier generations, the data collected were sent to physicians via the Internet to be interpreted, and thus detect anomalies and emergencies. With technological advancement, applications were developed to interpret and detect abnormal situations. These applications are implemented in the patient on a single computer, on touch pad or smart phone. If an anomaly is detected, these applications react accordingly, either by providing advice to the patient, or by calling an ambulance (depending on the level of the anomaly). The doctor in charge can track the state of his patients and receives alerts and anomalies detected.

In Part 2, we present generalities on ontologies and their advantages. Then in Section 3, we present some related work present in the literature, their advantages and inconveniences. Part 4 includes the proposal of a generic and adequate solution to the problem. Finally, we finish with a conclusion.

2. Ontologies

2.1. Definition

The first accepted definition for an ontology is that of [4], "explicit specification of a conceptualization".

This definition has also been recently clarified by [5] to be: "Ontology is an explicit formal specification and a shared conceptualization".

In this definition, it is necessary to correctly interpret each used term. Formal: the machine can understand. Explicit: the concepts, relationships, individuals and axioms are explicitly defined. Shared: knowledge representations are shared by a community. Conceptualization: abstract model of a part of the world that we want to represent.

2.2. Dimensions of classification

Ontologies can be classified along several dimensions. Among these, we focus on the typology based on the object of conceptualization.

Ontologies can be classified according to their conceptualization object as follows: Top level ontology, Domain ontology, Task ontology, Application ontology. As shown in Figure 1.

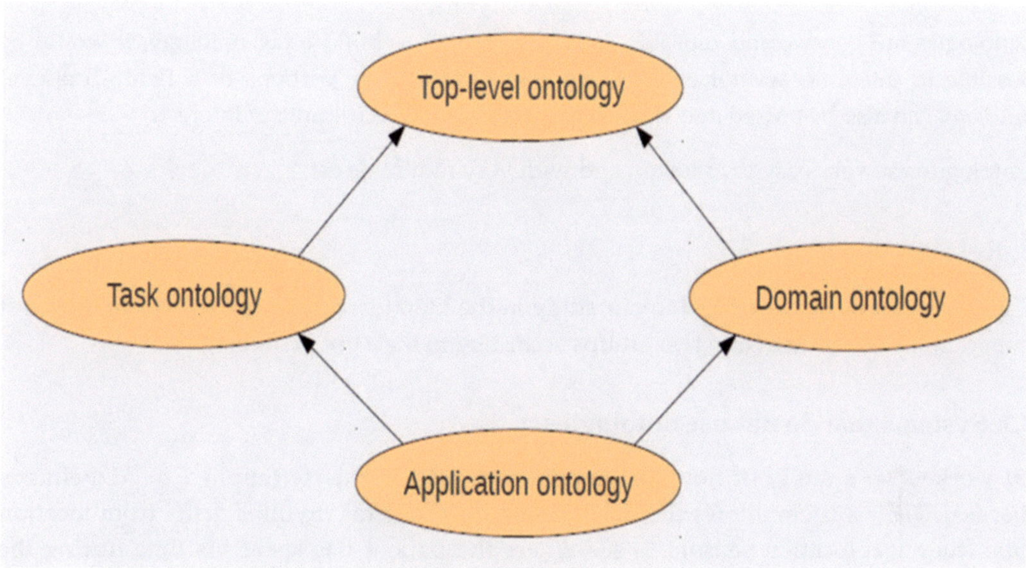

Figure 1. Classification of ontologies according to the object of conceptualization

Top level ontology [6], this type of ontology describes very general concepts or common sense knowledge such as space, time, event, action, etc. These concepts are independent of a problem or a particular area.

Domain ontology [7], this ontology governs a set of vocabularies and concepts describing an application domain or the target world. It characterizes the knowledge of the area where the task is performed. Most existing ontologies are domain ontologies.

Task ontology [7], this type of ontology is used to conceptualize specific tasks in systems. It governs a set of vocabularies and concepts describing a structure of performing the tasks domain-independent.

Application ontology [8], this ontology is the most specific. The concepts in the application ontology are very domain specific and particular application. In other words, the concepts often correspond to roles played by domain entities while performing a certain activity.

2.3. Contribution of ontologies

Ontologies provide a common semantics. This means that all individuals and concepts involved can be explicitly defined in terms of their relationships and attributes. Therefore, ontologies are interpreted by a machine and shared between several people. This facilitates and improves the quality of diagnosis and the process of decision support. Also, several people can work together without any ambiguity or loss of information.

Ontologies provide a model of high level abstraction of daily workflow. This model can be adapted to each organization. In other words, any organization can have an ontology adapted to its particular situation.

Ontologies are generic and reusable. If it is necessary to build a big ontology, it would be possible to integrate several existing ontologies describing portions of a field. Top-level ontology can also be reused and extended to describe a specific area of interest.

Ontologies are very easy to maintain and with very minimal cost.

3. Related work

There are a lot of works related to our study in the literature. We chose to present the most important dividing them into two groups according to their use of ontologies.

3.1. Systems that do not use ontologies

[9] worked on a study of home telemonitoring for the elderly (applied to Alzheimer's disease). Their system allows the detection of nycthemeral rhythms drifts from location data (they use location sensors to see where the patient has spent his time during the day). Recordings are made every second. Then one day measures are grouped by period of one hour or 15 minutes, to be compared by Hamming measure. Through this comparison, they can know when the patient slept and how many hours of sleep he had.

Other studies in the same context as [10-12] were made using sensors location of the patient. These studies are based on classification methods to analyze the patient's daily activities.

[13] propose a telemonitoring system with architecture of three levels: the sensor network, the patient server that collects and transmits the information, and the hospital server that processes information and makes them available to physicians. This system uses data mining to detect anomalies.

[14] worked on the project TISSAD which develops medical remote monitoring systems at home. These systems are designed for elderly and / or chronic conditions, to prevent accidents or aggravation of their health conditions. The system is based on the recovery of vital or behavioral data and saves them in a database. Then due to an intelligent module, it makes computer-aided diagnosis. The project TISSAD was centered on the user by consolidating data into four classes: identification, historical requirements, medical history and medical data.

[15] proposed a strategy to implement an alarm component in remote monitoring system of elderly people. The system consists of units in the homes of people monitored for collecting from sensors (medical and environmental) and sending data, and a call center with a server for recording and tracking data. Alerts are modeled in XML.

3.2. Limits of systems that do not use ontologies

Systems seen previously are based on old technologies. These technologies are characterized by the absence of semantics, which implies that the machine is not able to interpret the results. The lack of ontologies reduces their performance and making them difficult to share and evolve. In addition, they use data formats specific to them, making the information and data not generic and communication with other systems very complicated. The decision support is either lacking or based on data mining, or by using very complex processes.

For systems that do not provide decision support as those presented by [9, 12], despite that its systems are simple and not expensive, the machine cannot interpret data collected after their classification, specialists must monitor the activities of patients.

Using only data mining, the system will generate false alarms or will not detect anomalies due to the probabilistic characteristic of data mining. Errors will therefore introduce the facts base and will generate even more mistakes. This implies a degradation of system performance over time.

Without the use of ontologies, the inference process becomes very complex and difficult to change because the handled information is poorly structured so difficult to exploit. Also due to the characteristic "linked data" of ontologies, inference becomes easy and automatic as the use of transitivity, reflexivity, etc.

3.3. Systems using ontologies

[16] propose a system of decision support for remote monitoring of patients with heart failure. The system is based on an ontology which includes patient data: posture, pulse sensor, physical activities and alerts. The decision aid is based on inference using rules managed by an inference algorithm.

This system does not take into account physiological measures that are connected to the heart failure like blood pressure and weight data, nor the patient's environment such as temperature and humidity. Moreover, the context of the patient is very small for such physical activity as it contains statements: run, walk or anything, and also the posture he has only two states: lying or standing. Finally, the proposed inference algorithm is not optimal because a rule can have multiple conditions, for each condition the algorithm cover all the facts base, when he could have in some cases use the results of other conditions.

[17] propose a system based on multiple ontologies: the personal data of the patient, the context of the house (environment), social context (people connected to the patient) and alarms. The system uses the rule-based inference of first order, these rules are very dependent on the parameters (example: if temperature> 40 then alert) making them non generic and non-scalable. The rules do not take into account changes in health state of the patient. Moreover, the rules can change from one patient to another but it is done manually by experts implying important feedback.

[18] detail the design and implementation of a platform for reasoning to anticipate and react intelligently in situations demanding long-distance care or at home. The system manages intelligent agents, whose behavior is defined and validated by ontologies and rules. A development methodology has been adapted to support the process of knowledge acquisition. Log files are stored in XML to make data mining algorithms.

[19-21] proposed an ontological architecture for modeling a system Smart Home e-health. The goal is to provide an adaptive system for extending the home support of an aging person with diminished cognitive autonomy. The architecture is based on seven ontologies: housing, equipment, person, behavior, task, software application and the decision. These ontologies are interconnected.

3.4. Limits of presented systems using ontologies

These systems only partially integrate ontologies and do not contain domain ontologies that provide a controlled vocabulary standard to better share information and make it more generic.

In most cases, information about the patient are not fully exploited, each system is based on part of data (physiological, environmental, behavioral), although these data are strongly related and should be exploited in the same process to ensure decision support more accurate.

Moreover, the inference engines are based on rules defined by experts, but these rules are not scalable and do not take into account changes in health status of the patient. In the case where experts fail to mention a few cases and few rules, the system is unable to detect anomalies.

[22] Propose the most complete architecture in those studied. It consists of several ontologies for symptoms, diseases, medications, measures and patients. An inference engine on these ontologies. In addition, a status history of the patient and a history of actions taken are stored in another database. Methods of data mining are used on both historical to produce new rules that will supply a second inference engine. This inference engine has as facts base both historical.

This system is very complicated because it must handle ontologies and relational databases at the same time. This implies synchronization between the two bases, with a risk of loss of information and semantics. The use of two inference engines simultaneously reduces system performance in terms of response time.

4. Proposition

From systems seen previously, we will try to propose a general and generic architecture based on ontologies for telemonitoring of elderly person or person suffering from a chronic disease such as heart failure, kidney disease or Alzheimer's pathology.

This architecture is based on ontologies and decision support. The aim is to detect anomalies or dangerous situations by collecting physiological data (heart rhythms, temperature, weight, etc.) or behavioral (daily activities, posture, etc) about the patient as well as information from its environment (light, temperature, humidity, magnetic field, etc).

This architecture is shown in *figure 2* and consists of several parts with two principal actors who are medical experts and system experts. The architecture contains two types of ontologies:

- The ontology that manages the system (users, sensors, measurements, alarms, etc). We call this ontology "application ontology". The architecture of this ontology is defined by the system specifications.
- The domain ontologies are used to define a controlled vocabulary (diseases, medications, symptoms, etc). These ontologies are connected to the application ontology and will complete it by defining some of its concepts. These ontologies are built by medical experts.

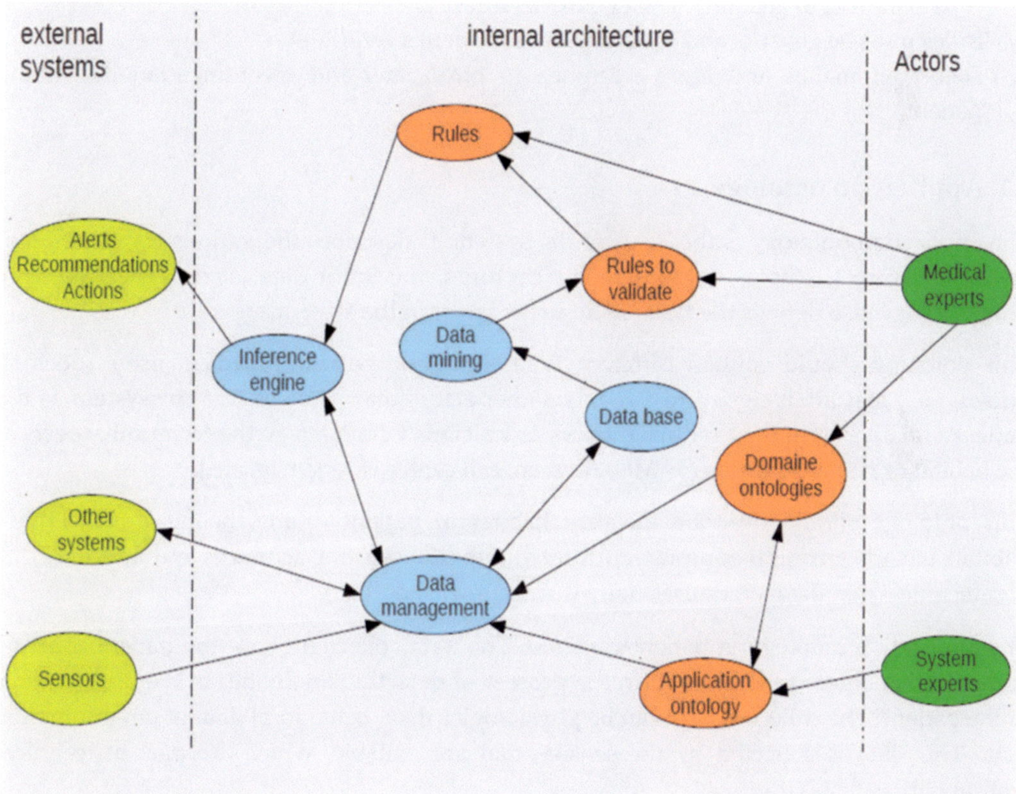

Figure 2. System Architecture

The decision support is based on an inference engine that receives as input the rules of inference and the facts that is provided by the *"data management"* part. The rules are introduced either by medical experts, or generated by a data mining then validated by medical experts. The inference engine detects anomalies and raises alerts informing doctors.

- Data Management part is the core of the system, its main features are:
- Receive data from sensors.
- Communicate with other systems.
- Provide a facts base for the inference engine and receive the data inferred.
- Manage the database and ontologies.
- Our system must meet the following requirements:
- It must cover all patient information (physiological, environmental, behavioral), and represent them to facilitate the detection of abnormalities and dangerous situation.
- It must contain a controlled vocabulary to communicate unambiguously with other systems.
- The solution should be generic and can be used for any system of medical monitoring.
- Collect patient data from sensors or doctors and store them.
- Infer the state of the patient based on his background and the data collected and the rules defined by medical experts.
- A data mining to generate new evolutives rules.
- Rules must be generic, and evolve with the patient's condition.
- Detect anomalies and issue warnings to physicians and recommendations for the patient.

4.1. Application ontology

The application ontology is the heart of the system. It describes the various components of the system (users, sensors, measurements captured, the input data, alerts generated, etc). This ontology also defines the tasks of different actors in the system.

This ontology should contain different types of users, patients, medical users (doctors, nurses, etc.) that are assigned to patients. Other actors may have to use our system as the patient's relatives (families and neighbors), technicians who manage the technical aspects of the habitat or response teams (SAMU, firemen, call center emergency, etc.).

This ontology should describe the care habitat of patient (home, hospital, etc.). These habitats include technical equipment (different types of sensors, actuators and machines), or non-technical that the patient uses daily (furniture, dishes, etc.).

The application ontology is patient-centered. The data collected about the patient must be stored in this ontology to be used in the process of detecting anomalies in the health status of the patient. The collected data can be physiologies data, behavioral data or environmental data. This data is collected by the sensors that are suitable, which are part of technical equipment.

4.2. Domain ontologies

The domain ontologies aim to complete the application ontology by providing a controlled vocabulary, as for diseases, symptoms and medications. These ontologies can provide a language for sharing and communication between different actors in the system. With the semantics of these ontologies, our system can interact easily with other systems. Thus, data and information processed are generic and can be introduced into other systems.

These ontologies are built by medical experts, aided by knowledge engineers to formalize them. These ontologies can be linked between them, for example, link disease to symptoms.

We can also construct ontology from a medical corpus made up of stories, publications, regulations, etc. With text mining techniques applied on this corpus, we define a controlled vocabulary. This controlled vocabulary is transformed into ontology by creating relationships between different terms such as the relationship of hierarchy.

We can also use controlled vocabularies existing in literature and transform them into ontologies. [23] use this method to build two ontologies, one for diseases and the second for the symptoms.

Due to the reusability of ontologies, ontologies existing in literature can be reused as the one built by [23, 24].

4.3. Decision support

The decision support is reflected in the detection of abnormalities and changes in health status of the patient. It is ensured by an inference engine based on rules. These rules should be as generic as possible, and must evolve with the patient's state.

Inferred data provide recommendations and advice to the patient if necessary. If abnormal conditions are detected, in this case, the system must send alerts to the medical staff or the patient's family or his neighbors, or in an emergency, the call center and teams intervention. They can also lead to an action on the machines and actuators in the habitat. Inferred data can help the doctor diagnose the patient by providing information of the evolution of his health.

The rules are defined by medical experts and can change over time. Rules can also be generated after a data mining done on the databases. As data mining is probabilistic, rules must be validated by medical experts.

For each new event (data collection), the inference engine is started to try to apply the rules of this new data. If new data is generated by the inference engine, then resume the process from start, taking the new data as new events. This process stops when there are no rules to fire or that rules do not generate new knowledge.

5. Conclusion

In this paper we proposed a solution for managing data and detect anomalies in a telemonitoring system.

Telemonitoring systems are based on the collection of information from physiologies, environmental or behavioral sensors. In the first systems, these data were interpreted by physicians directly. But with technological advancement, expert systems have been developed for the automatic processing of data.

We studied various proposals and solutions existing in literature and we presented the most important.

We proposed a general solution that relies on the use of different types of ontologies, an ontology management system, and domain ontologies.

Using ontologies, this solution is generic, sharable and can communicate with other systems without ambiguities.

This solution is based on inference to detect anomalies and changes in patient's state. This inference is based on rules that are defined by medical experts or generated by a data mining followed by a validation by medical experts.

Author details

Amine Ahmed Benyahia
Université de Technologie Belfort-Montbéliard, Belfort, France
NEWEL, Mulhouse, France

Amir Hajjam and Vincent Hilaire
Université de Technologie Belfort-Montbéliard, Belfort, France

Mohamed Hajjam
NEWEL, Mulhouse, France

6. References

[1] Pierre Barralon. 2005. Classification et fusion de données actimétriques pour la télésurveillance médicale. Projet de thèse, université Joseph Fourier.
[2] La telesante : un nouvel atout au service de notre bien-être : Un plan quinquennal éco-responsable pour le déploiement de la télésanté en France.(2009), Rapport remis à Madame Roselyne Bachelot-Narquin, Ministre de la Santé et des Sports par Monsieur Pierre Lasbordes, Député de l'Essonne.
[3] Agostino Giorgio. 2011. Innovative Medical Devices for Telemedicine Applications. In Telemedicine Techniques and Applications, Edited by Georgi Graschew and Stefan Rakowsky, pp 19-44.
[4] T. Gruber, 2003. Towards principals for the design of ontologies used for knowledge sharing. Formal ontology in conceptual analysis and knowledge representation. Kluwer Academic pubishers.
[5] Studer Benjamins Fensel. 1998. Knowledge Engeenering : Principles and Methods. Data and Knowledge Engineering 25, 161-197
[6] J. Sowa. 1995. Top-level ontological categories. International Journal of Human and Computer Studies, 43, 669-685.

[7] R. Mizoguchi, K. Kozaki, T. Sano et Y. Kitamura 2000. Construction and Deployment of a Plant Ontology. The 12th International Conference, EKAW2000, 113-128.

[8] A. Maedche. 2002. Ontology Learning for the Semantic Web. Boston: Kluwer Academic Publishers.

[9] C. Franco, J. Demongeot, C. Villemazet , N. Vuillerme. 2010. Behavioral telemonitoring of the elderly at home : Detection of nycthemeral rhythms drifts from location data. 24th International Conference on Advanced Information Networking and Applications Workshops, 759-766.

[10] Tareq Hadidi, Norbert Noury. 2009. A Predictive Analysis of the Night-Day Activities Level of Older Patient in a Health Smart Home. Ambient Assistive Health and Wellness Management in the Heart of the City. 290-293

[11] C. Franco, J. Demongeot, Y. Fouquet, C. Villemazet, N. Vuillerme. 2010. Perspectives in home TeleHealthCare system: Daily routine nycthemeral rhythm monitoring from location data. International Conference on Complex, Intelligent and Software Intensive Systems. 611-617.

[12] Anthony Fleury, Michel Vacher, Norbert Noury. 2010. SVM-Based Multi-Modal Classification of Activities of Daily Living in Health Smart Homes: Sensors, Algorithms and First Experimental Results. IEEE TRANSACTION ON INFORMATION TECHNOLOGY IN BIOMEDICINE. 274-283.

[13] Rifat Shahriyar, Md. Faizul Bari, Gourab Kundu, Sheikh Iqbal Ahamed, and Md. Mostofa Akbar. 2009. Intelligent Mobile Health Monitoring System (IMHMS). International Journal of Control and Automation, Vol.2, No.3, 13-28.

[14] Jean-Pierre Thomesse et l'équipe du projet TIISSAD. 2002. Les technologies de l'information intégrées aux services de soin à domicile : Le projet TIISSAD. Informatique et santé, 27-34.

[15] V. Stoicu-Tivadar , L. Stoicu-Tivadar , V.Topac and D. Berian. 2009. A WebService-based Alarm Solution in a TeleCare System. 5th International Symposium on Applied Computational Intelligence and Informatics. 117-121.

[16] Aniello Minutolo, Giovanna Sannino, Massimo Esposito, Giuseppe De Pietro. 2010. A rule-based mHealth system for cardiac monitoring. 2010 IEEE EMBS Conference on Biomedical Engineering & Sciences.

[17] Federica Paganelli, Dino Giuli. 2011. An Ontology-Based System for Context-Aware and Configurable Services to Support Home-Based Continuous Care. IEEE TRANSACTIONS ON INFORMATION TECHNOLOGY IN BIOMEDICINE, VOL. 15, NO. 2, MARCH 2011.

[18] Miguel A. Valero, Laura Vadillo, Iván Pau, and Ana Peñalver. 2009. An Intelligent Agents Reasoning Platform to Support Smart Home Telecare. IWANN 2009, Part II, LNCS 5518. 679–686.

[19] F. Latfi, B. Lefebvre and C. Descheneaux. 2007. Le rôle de l'ontologie de la tâche dans un Habitat Intelligent en Télé-Santé. 1ères Journées Francophones sur les Ontologies JFO, Sousse, Tunisie, 18 - 20 Octobre 2007.

[20] F. Latfi, C. Descheneaux, B. Lefebvre. 2007. Habitat intelligent en télé–Santé : ontologie de l'équipement. FICCDAT, 16-19 Juin. Toronto, Canada, 2007.

[21] F. Latfi, B. Lefebvre, C. Descheneaux. 2007. Ontology-based management of the telehealth smart home, dedicated to elderly in loss of cognitive autonomy , OWLED 2007. June 6-7 Innsbruck, Austria.

[22] Rocio Martinez-Lopez, David Millan-Ruiz, Alberto Martin-Dominguez, Maria Aranzazu Toro-Escudero. 2008. An architecture for Next-generation of Telecare Systems using ontologies. Rules Engines and Data Mining.

[23] T.A Gavrilova, R.A Ravodin, E.S. Bolotnikova. 2011. Development of Dermatovenereology Ontology for Education and Expert Support.

[24] B.E. Dixon, A. Zafar, J.J. McGowan. (2007), Development of a Taxonomy for Health Information Technology, in K. A. Kuhn, J. R. Warren & T.-Y. Leong, eds, 'Proceedings of the 12th World Congress on Health (Medical) Informatics, MEDINFO 2007', Vol. 129 of Studies in Health Technology and Informatics, IOS Press, Brisbane, Australia, pp. 616–620.

Chapter 6

Advances and Perspectives in the Field of Auscultation, with a Special Focus on the Contribution of New Intelligent Communicating Stethoscope Systems in Clinical Practice, in Teaching and Telemedicine

Emmanuel Andrès

Additional information is available at the end of the chapter

http://dx.doi.org/10.5772/48402

1. Introduction

The stethoscope and the semantic of auscultatory findings were invented more than 200 years ago by Dr. Laennec (*Traité de l'Auscultation Médiate*, Paris, 1819 [**Figure 1**]) and over the years very few changes have been made to both the stethoscope itself and the way in which it is used [1]. However, the ability to differentiate between normal and abnormal sounds or noises (vesicular sounds, wheezes, crackles, etc) remains essential in clinical practice for correct diagnosis and management.

Over the past two decades, much of the progress made in this area has resulted primarily from improvements made to the stethoscope itself [1]. More recently, we have seen advances in the techniques used to process auscultatory signals as well as in the analysis and clarification of the resulting sounds [2,3]. The availability of novel representations of the sounds, with phono- and spectrograms, also opens interesting perspectives in the context of diagnostic aids, but also in education and pedagogy [4].

This chapter aims to review recent technological advances, evaluate promising innovations and perspectives in the field of auscultation, with a special focus on the development of new intelligent communicating stethoscope systems in clinical practice, and in the context of teaching and telemedicine.

2. Current semantic of auscultatory findings and characterization of sounds

The physical characterization of physiological and pathological sounds in humans is still at a fledgling stage and has not yet resulted in reliable documentation, especially not so in the field of pulmonary auscultation [2]. In cardiology, the situation is somewhat similar. However, more precise data, essentially based on phonocardiography, are available, outdated as they may be [1]. Analysis and characterization of auscultation sounds have been totally neglected by practicing physicians and any major improvements have been made were primarily in auscultatory tools, i.e., the new intelligent communicating stethoscope systems [4].

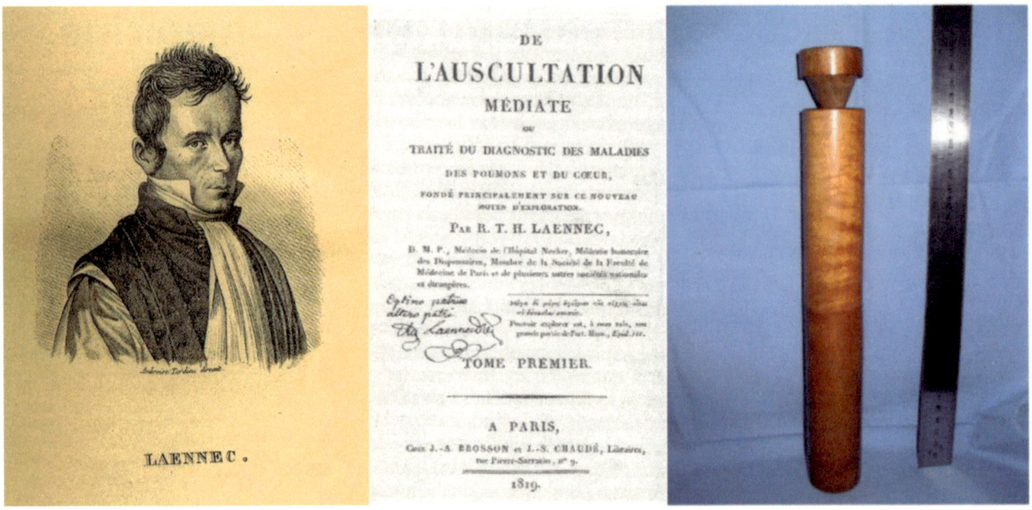

Figure 1. Portrait of René Théophile Hyacinthe Laennec. Front cover of the first edition of the *"Traité de l'Auscultation Médiate"*, Paris, France, 1819. Note the handwritten Latin dedication to his uncle Guillaume Laennec in Nantes: *"A mon excellent oncle, mon autre père"* ("To my great uncle, my other father"). The original Laennec stethoscope, in wood, retains in the Museum of the History of Medicine, in Paris, France.

Whilst conventional stethoscope auscultation is subjective and hardly sharable, the characterization and identification of sounds by computer-based recording and analysis systems provide objective and early diagnostic help along with better sensitivity and reproducibility [2]. The precise definition of these physical characteristics and the availability of new visual representations of sounds constitute exciting perspectives for teaching and pedagogy, as we shall see later in this chapter [5].

Thus, as we have hypothesized, the new intelligent communicating stethoscope systems will also possibly contribute to a new auscultatory semiology, based on reliable methods of signal analysis and on visual display, and will be complementary to the acoustic signals perceived by the practitioner [2,6].

Breath sounds or noises are produced by airflow in the respiratory system as well as the work of the breathing apparatus. These sounds are characterized by a wide spectrum of different sounds - the average frequency depends on the site of auscultation [**3**]. It is generally accepted that the frequency of lung sounds ranges between 50 and 2500 Hz, while tracheal sounds can reach up to 4000 Hz [2,3,5]. In terms of respiratory pathology, it should be emphasized that, only a small number of sounds are currently well identified and documented in regard of physical characteristics (*for review see the reference* [2]).

Table 1 gives a description of various auscultatory findings - normal breath sound, namely the vesicular murmur, and abnormal (pathological) - use clinically according to international literature [3,4].

Type of lung sounds according to international nomenclature	**Clinical Features**	**Pathological circumstances**
Vesicular murmur	Very soft noise, audible throughout the entire phase of inspiration and during early expiration. Detected in antero-lateral areas of the chest and in the back, it consists in a continuous, soft low intensity murmur, heard throughout inspiration	The vesicular murmur is weakened in the following circumstances: - extensive thickening of the wall, for example, in obesity), for example, in cases of emphysema (chest hyperinflation. It is abolished when : - the lung is collapsed by the pressure of fluid or air in the pleural cavity, such as in cases of pneumothorax or pleurisy - absence of ventilation in the affected lung area, for example, in cases of lung compression, especially in atelectasis with retraction - after pneumonectomy, on the operated side.
Wheezes and whistles	Of bronchial origin and variable intensity, wheezes are heard at a distance from the patient. They include inspiratory wheezes, as well as sibilant wheezes heard during both phases of breathing.	In cases of localized wheezing, it can be heard during inspiration or during both phases, with similar pitch, caused by partial obstruction of the trachea or bronchi, due to the presence of a tumor or foreign body. In cases of diffuse wheezing, it is most often in the form of bilateral wheezing, of various tonalities, heard especially at the end of expiration and encountered in instances of bronchial asthma. In chronic obstructive bronchitis (bronchial pneumonia), there is also diffuse expiratory wheezing, due to vibration of the bronchial walls which tend to collapse at expiration.
Rhonchi or snoring	Also of bronchial origin, sonorous rhonchi are low-pitched, in both inspiratory and expiratory phases, and altered by coughing.	They are encountered in acute or chronic bronchitis accompanied with bronchial hypersecretion. Usually cleared by coughing, the so-called fixed rhonchus on the other hand does not disappear after coughing effort and is generally associated with downstream bronchial obstruction.
Coarse crackles (or rales)	Also called mucous rales, bubbling rales are discontinuous and of short duration. Emitted sounds are irregular, uneven, intense, observed in both phases of respiration and altered by coughing.	They make a gurgling noise in the large airways often associated with bronchial congestion due to hypersecretion of mucus. They are predominantly observed in bronchitis.

Type of lung sounds according to international nomenclature	Clinical Features	Pathological circumstances
Fine crackles (or rales)	Also called fine rales or crepitations, they emit discontinuous, thin, dry noises, high and evenly pitched, occurring in spells during inspiration.	They become more distinctive after coughing and usually point to an alveolar disease process. Due to alveolar wall detachment and their pathological features, they are observed primarily in cases of pneumonia, interstitial alveolar or pulmonary edema subsequent to heart failure, but also in pulmonary fibrosis and in certain interstitial pneumonias.
Bronchial or tubular breathing Bronchial sound	A coarse, high intensity and high-pitch noise that can be heard in both inspiratory and expiratory phases, although predominantly inspiratory.	It can be heard over the thorax suggesting pneumonia-induced pulmonary consolidation and is typically accompanied by a series of crackles
Pleural breathing sound	A soft, distant, veiled expiratory sound.	It is heard at the upper limit of moderate pleural effusion. Like (bronchial or tubular) breathing, it is determined by pulmonary consolidation complicated by pleurisy. Although attenuated by the latter, it nevertheless exhibits different features than (bronchial, tubular) breathing.
Amphoric breathing	A high-pitch expiratory metallic sound	It is caused by the resonance of normal breath sounds in an air pocket, for example in cases of pneumothorax (with a persistent pleural breach).
Pleural rub or Pleural friction rub	Dry grating and superficial sounds, unchanged by coughing. Their Intensity may be discrete, like the «rustle of silk paper», or intense, such as the «creaking sound of new leather».	They are due to the two inflamed pleural layers rubbing against each other. They occur at the onset of pleurisy, at its upper limit or after fluid evacuation. The differential diagnosis with that of coarse crackles may be difficult, but unlike the latter, pleural rubs appear soon after the start of inspiration.

Table 1. International semantic on normal and abnormal lung sounds use in clinical practice [2,7,8].

The generation of heart sounds is essentially related to cardiac muscle contraction, the functioning of the valves and turbulence generated by blood flow. The spectrum of heart sounds is between 20 and 100 Hz for baseline signals and higher frequencies for murmurs: 500 Hz and above [1,2]. S1, corresponding to the closure of the mitral and tricuspid valves, incorporate frequencies ranging from 10 to 100 Hz. S2, resulting from the opening of the aortic and pulmonary sigmoid valves, is of higher frequency, generally between 150 and 200 Hz. It should be noted that additional heart sounds (S3 and S4) may be heard and additional diastolic noises originating from the valves can also be observed with mitral opening snap, pericardial (friction) rub or knock, etc. Lastly, we can also detect so-called "organic murmurs" which are related to alterations of the mitral or tricuspid atrioventricular valves (inlet valves) or ventriculo-aortic or pulmonary valves (ejection valves) (*for review see the reference* [4]).

Figure 2 depicts the chronological and morphological characteristics of heart murmurs, illustrating how the practitioner makes a diagnosis by taking into account these elements when analyzing the auscultatory signal perceived [2].

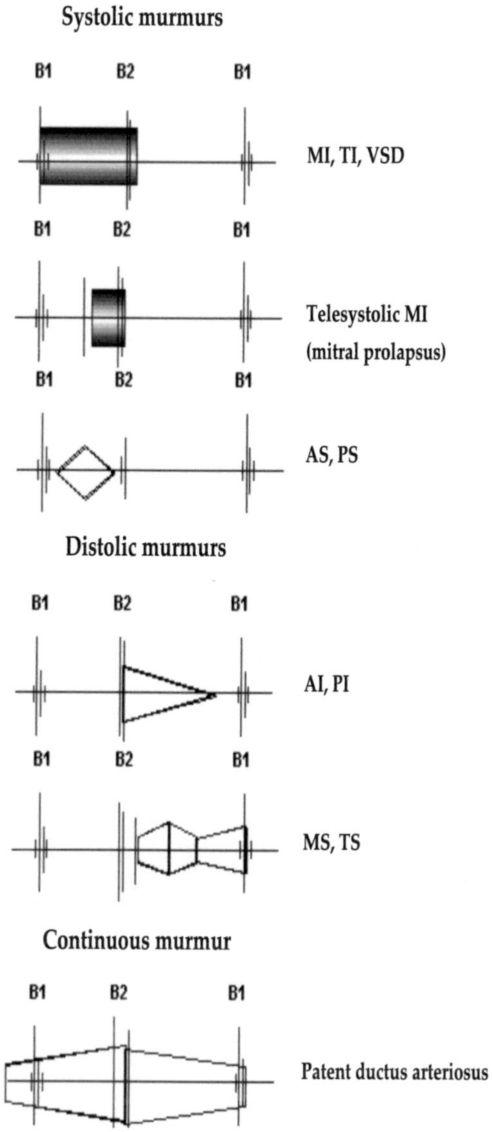

AS : aortic stenosis; AI : aortic insufficiency; PS : pulmonary stenosis; PI : pulmonary insufficiency; MS : mitral stenosis; MI : mitral insufficiency; TI: tricuspid insufficiency; TS : tricuspid stenosis; VSD : ventricular septal defect.

Figure 2. Schematic representation of breaths during the cardiac cycle.

3. Advances and perspectives in documentation and characterization of sounds

In practice, auscultation diagnoses are often made based solely on past experience of the practitioners, and rely more on intuition than on rigorous and systematic classification systems [1]. However in recent years, various studies have endeavored to characterize, identify and describe sounds in greater detail, especially in the respiratory field [5-8].

It is in this context that an innovative project known as ASAP: "*Analyse de Sons Auscultatoires et Pathologiques*" (Analysis of Auscultatory and Pathological Sounds) was developed by the French national agency for research (ANR 2006 - TLOG 21 04, headed by Professor E. Andrès) [5]. This project was supported by the development and the provision of a new intelligent communicating stethoscope system.

The main objective of this project was to bring pulmonary auscultation into the era of evidence-based medicine, based on the identification of sounds using innovations in technology, mathematics and computer science in order to "rediscover" the clinical significance of respiratory sounds [5]. The ASAP project allowed us to documented physically characterized these sounds in more detail.

To date, we have collected over 500 auscultations, well-documented clinically (**Figure 3**), and began an analysis of its physical characteristics of the sounds. Thus, physically-speaking, crackles correspond to a characteristic wave whose appearance is shown in **Figure 4**, a representation revisited and detailed elsewhere [4,9]. Note that it is generally accepted that the duration of crackles is less than 20 ms and their frequency is between 100 and 200 Hz [10]. A sibilant wheeze, on the other hand, is characterized by a waveform with a

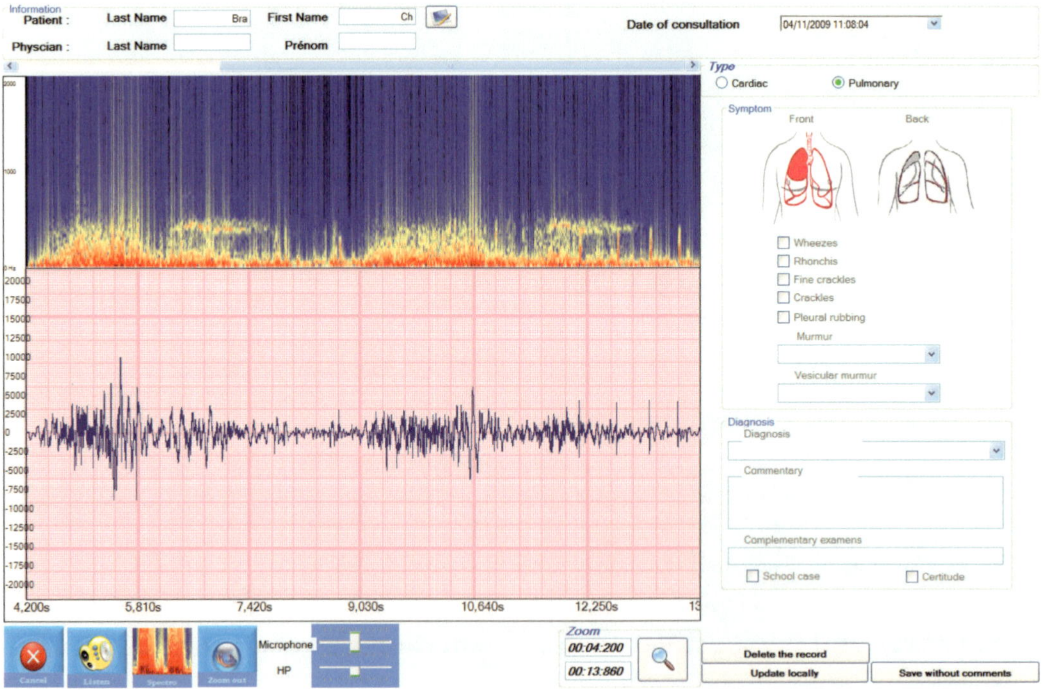

Figure 3. Clinical documentation and physical characterization of sounds collected through the ASAP project. These data includes: characteristics of the patient; auscultation type; acoustic data; diagnosis; sounds (*data collected in the ASAP project*) [5].

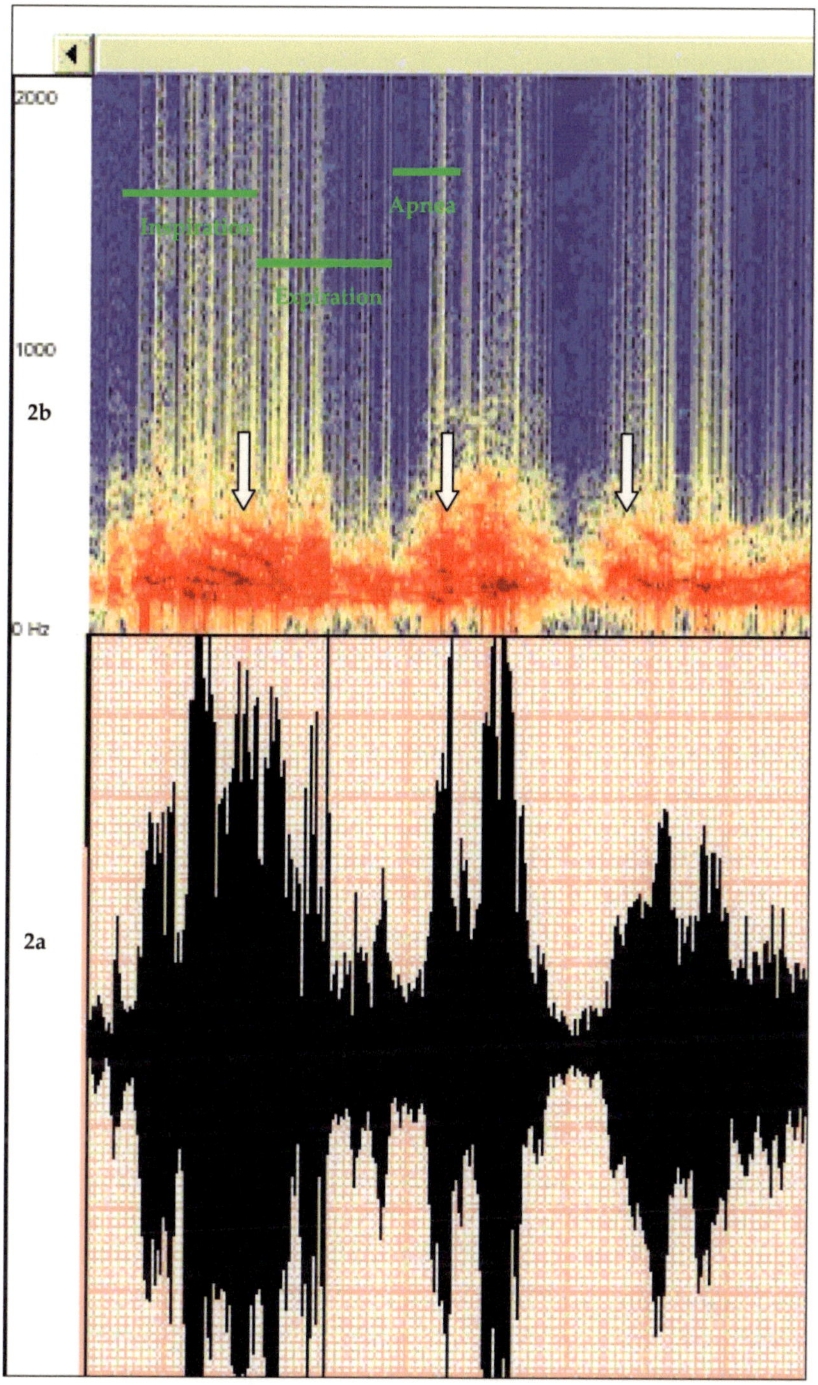

Figure 4. Representation of a breathing cycle in a patient with chronic obstructive pulmonary disease, along with respective phases of inspiration, expiration and respiratory pause in the form of a phonopneumogram (2a) and a spectrogram (2b). Presence of numerous coarse crackles especially visible on the spectrogram (2b) (indicated by arrows) (*data collected in the ASAP project*) [5].

dominant frequency usually above 100 Hz and a duration exceeding 100 ms. In terms of physics, wheezing sounds are longer than 50 or 100 ms but less than 250 ms [4,9,10]. The frequency of wheezes ranges between 100 and 2500 Hz with a characteristic peak frequency of 100 or 400 Hz and 1000 or 1600 Hz.

The ASAP project is complementary to other work conducted locally at the University Hospital (CHRU) of Strasbourg in collaboration with the research team led by Doctor C. Brandt, notably the project: *"Perspectives et apports du développement d'un stéthoscope communiquant à l'ère de la telemedicine"* (Perspectives and contributions of the development of a communicating stethoscope in the era of telemedicine) (PRI HUS - No. 4179, headed by Doctor C. Brandt and Professor E. Andrès, Strasbourg, France) [6].

The objectives of this project were: validation of a new communicating stethoscope we have developed (*see a next section of this chapter*); comparison of conventional (acoustic) auscultation with this new communicating stethoscope system; creating an auscultatory library; and development of expert systems for real-time analysis of signals from cardiovascular and pulmonary auscultation for diagnosis assistance.

Forward, the ASAP and PRI projects aims at making evolve the auscultation technics:

- first, by the development objective tools for the analyse of auscultation sounds: electronic stethoscopes paired with computing device;
- by the creation of an auscultation sounds' database in order to compare and identify the physical characteristics, the acoustical and visual signatures of the pathologies;
- and lastly, by the capitalisation of these new auscultation techniques around the creation of a teaching unit and a school of auscultation on the *web* (*http://www.websound.fr*) [5,6]. This auscultation's school, potentially hosted on the *web*, will be destined to the initial and continuous formation of the medical attendants (**Figure 5**).

4. Advances in the field of sound representation and perspectives in teaching

Whereas conventional auscultation is subjective and interpreted by a single clinician, the characterization of sounds through recording, analysis and auscultatory signal processing systems provides in several studies better sensitivity and specificity when interpreting findings [4,11]. The availability of new technologies opens up interesting perspectives in the field of diagnostic tools, but also in education [4,12].

In fact, as well as providing a reliable addition to routine clinical diagnosis, these "tools" should ultimately lead to improvements in auscultatory training, based on the "physical" characterization of signals and sounds, as well as a visual representation in the form of:

- phonopneumogram or phonocardiogram: a tool providing simultaneous representation in time of the respiratory phases (**Figure 2a**) or the cardiac cycle and the auscultation signal (**Figure 6a**);

- spectrogram: a tool where time is indicated on the abscissa, frequency on the ordinate and the intensity of the signal is represented by a color palette for the respiratory *(Figure 2b)* or heart signal *(**Figure 6b**)*.

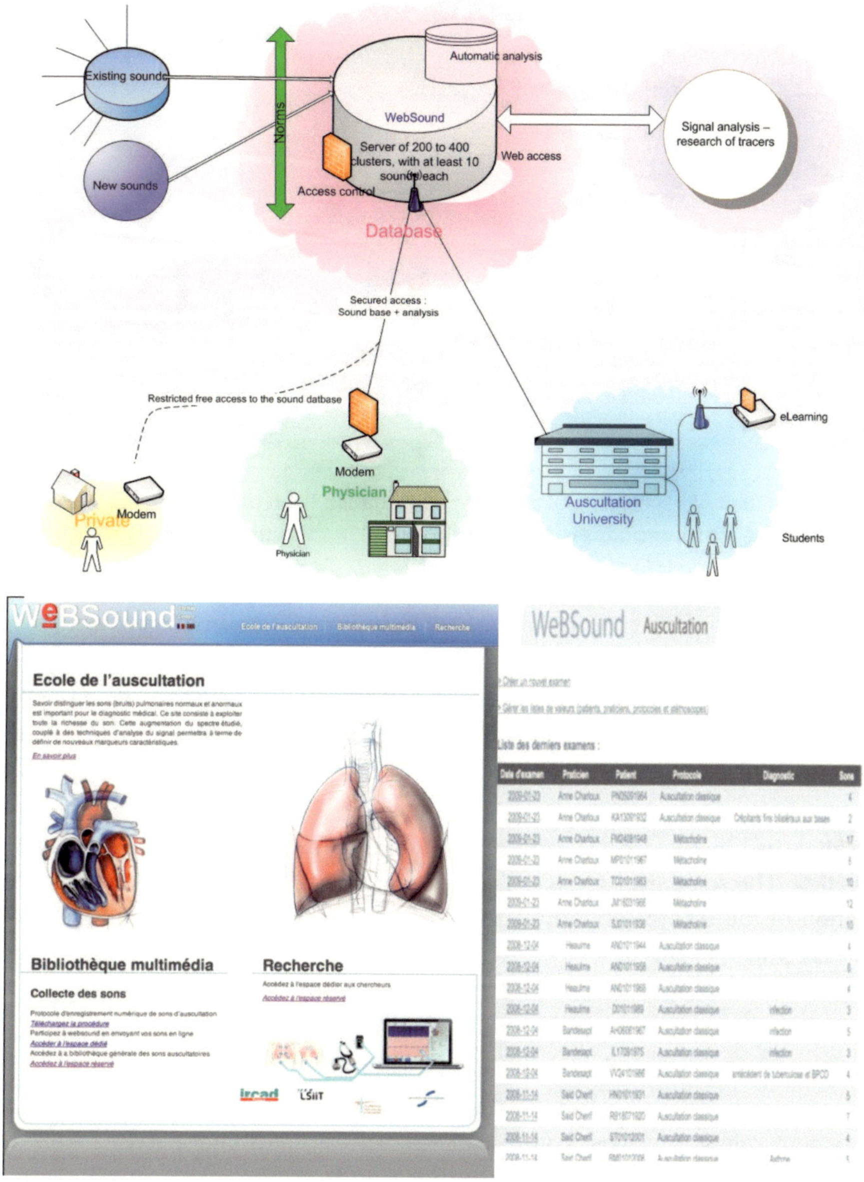

Figure 5. Potential teaching contributions of advances and innovations in the field of auscultation with the creation of a school of auscultation on the web [4,5]. This school of auscultation includes several components: Patient follow-up, Collection of sounds, Consultation, Transmission, Listening, Analysis, Validated and classified respiratory sounds, Automated analysis, Sound database, Secured access, Students, Initial training, School of Auscultation, Physicians, Diagnostic aid, Continuing Education, Specialists, Certification Validation.

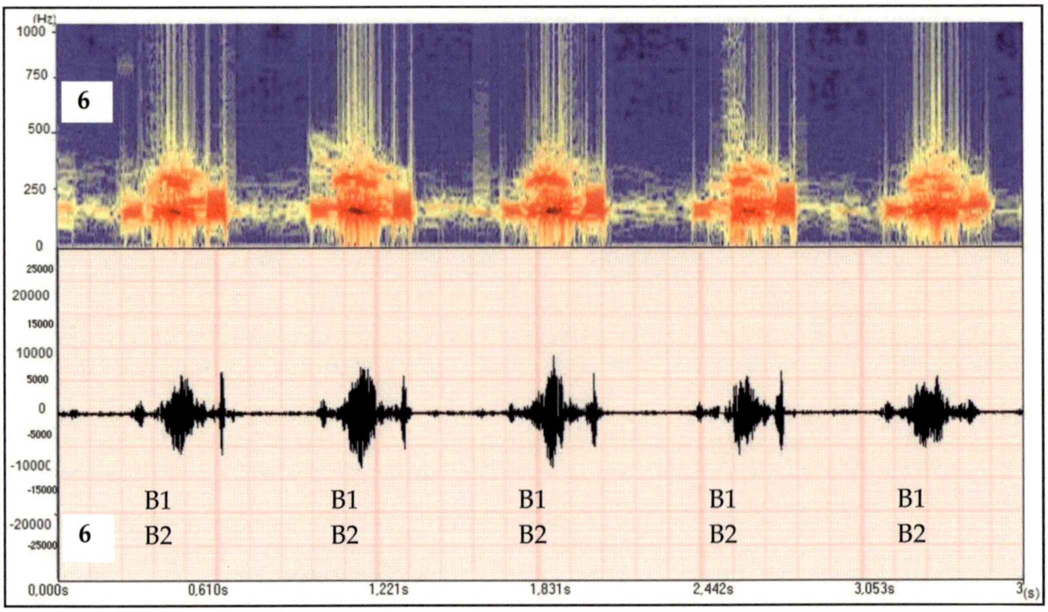

Figure 6. Representation of a recording of a cardiac auscultation in an individual with aortic stenosis with a systolic ejection murmur (indicated by a white arrow) in the form of a phonocardiogram (6a) and a spectrogram (6b) (*data collected in the PRI project*) [4,5].

To have a sort of proof of concept of the *"plus value"* of our intelligent communicating stethoscope system, we conducted a preliminary study at the University Hospital of Strasbourg with the aim of evaluating the diagnostic "performance" of these new visualization tools (phono- and spectrogram). We asked a cohort of medical graduate students (n = 30) to listen to 10 sounds in order to diagnose heart and lung pathology [13].

They were then asked to tick the appropriate box corresponding to the diagnosis relating to the sound they had just heard (as with an acoustic stethoscope). The correct response rate was 40 to 60 %. The same exercise was then carried out again with the addition of a visual representation of the sound (phonopneumogram or phonocardiogram and spectrograms). In this second phase of the trial, the rate of correct diagnosis reached 70 to 90%. **Table 2** presents the detail of these data. Analysis of this table shows that the improved performance (rate of correct diagnosis) is particularly significant for cardiac pathology.

Thus in our experience, addition of visual representation of sounds has significant implications in terms of medical medical education, and also in term of decision-making, potential patient safety, and cost control. In the field of teaching, a recent well designed study conducted by Sestini *et al.* supports the results of our work, concluding that an association between the acoustic signal and the image is highly useful for learning and understanding the basis of respiratory sounds [12].

To date, several stethoscopes on the market are already accompanied by specialized software providing the physician with a "visual representation of sounds", using various time-frequency representations, in the form of images. These can then be used in conjunction with the auditory information obtained from a stethoscope to achieve a diagnosis [6]. This "second channel" of information allows the practitioner to strengthen his clinical findings, and is likely to result in a more reliable diagnosis [14]. **Figure 7** illustrates this concept by using the example of aortic insufficiency (confirmed by cardiac ultrasound scan) which was not heard with the acoustic stethoscope but was visualized using our intelligent stethoscope prototype from the ASAP project [4]. This is a major achievement, using advances in medical technology to facilitate the work and training of practitioners.

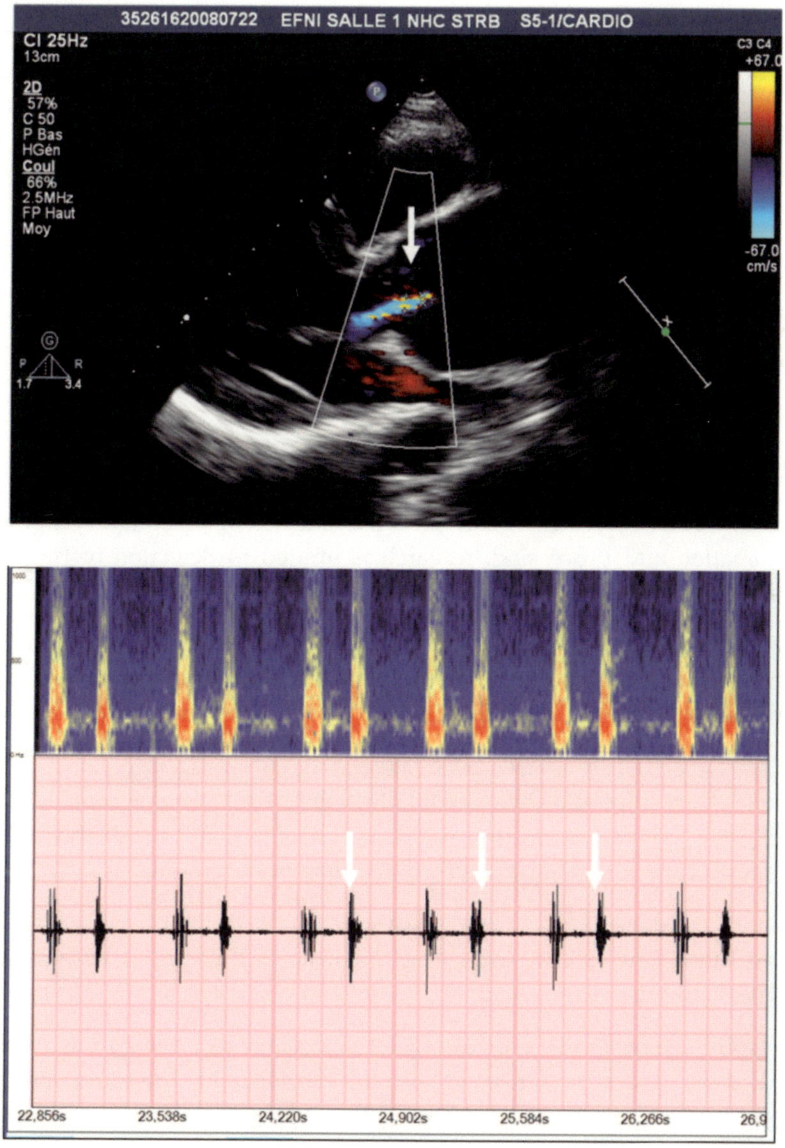

Figure 7. Aortic insufficiency (indicated by white arrows) not heard with the acoustic stethoscope but visualized using our intelligent stethoscope prototype and confirmed by echocardiography (*data collected in the ASAP project*) [4].

	All students (n = 30)	
	Without tools	With tools
% of "good" diagnosis (n = 10)	64% (191)	80% (239)
% of "good" diagnosis in respiratory auscultation (n = 5):	61% (92)	70% (105)
normal respiratory auscultation	57% (17)	63% (19)
crackles (chronic bronchitis)	57% (17)	60% (18)
crackles (interstitial pneumonia)	53% (16)	70% (21)
wheeze sibilants (acute crisis of asthma)	70% (21)	83% (25)
stridor (lung carcinoma)	70% (21)	73% (22)
% of "good" diagnosis in cardiac auscultation (n = 5):	66% (99)	89% (134)
normal cardiac auscultation	73% (22)	93% (28)
aortic stenosis	60% (18)	100% (30)
aortic regurgitation (minimal murmur)	30% (30)	70% (21)
mitral stenosis	40% (12)	87% (26)
arrhythmia (auricular fibrillation)	57% (17)	97% (29)

Table 2. Results of the use of new tools as phono- and spectrogram for visualizing sounds in 30 medical students [13].

5. Advances and innovations in the field of auscultatory signal analysis

To date, there has been very little research on the analysis of auscultatory signals. In terms of signal automation and processing, research is limited to detection of frequency peaks, sound duration measurements, etc [15,16].

In cardiology, little work has been conducted to render the stethoscope "intelligent" by allowing it to provide the clinician with an advanced diagnostic tool, as, for example, that provided by ECG systems which offer the practitioner a plot analysis as a diagnostic aid [14,17].

Of note is the work by Mint and Dillard who developed a stethoscope capable of diagnosing systolic or diastolic sounds present between B1 and B2 beats, and which measured the heart rate using a simple time-frequency analysis of the time periods of interest [14].

We also should acknowledge the work carried out by Murphy, who worked towards developing an "intelligent" stethoscope for which the technology is both interesting and innovative. These studies are reviewed, appended and presented in detail in reference [2].

In terms of respiratory medicine, the automated analysis of pulmonary auscultatory signals remains a challenge, especially compared with the cardiac field. The European Community-funded CORSA project, conducted between 1990 and 2000, provides an overview of the technical advances in respiratory sound analysis using signal processing tools [8,18].

Several studies have also provided an update on the various techniques used for the capture and digitization of respiratory sounds as well as giving an overview of analytical methods based on more standardized semantics [17-20]. A summary of the techniques and characteristics of the leading methods used to assess each type of respiratory sound is provided in references [2,16,17].

As part of the ASAP project mentioned above [5], the team led by Professor C. Collet of the Image Sciences, Computer Sciences and Remote Sensing Laboratory (LSIIT) of the University of Strasbourg (in Strasbourg, France), developed a novel approach in automated analysis of pulmonary auscultation signals [20-22]. As a second step, we then validated this approach on a small number of patients presenting with either: an auscultation defined as "normal", COPD with numerous crackles or asthma with wheezing.

The methods developed by C. Collet's team involve multiresolution signal analysis through the use of Bayesian tools in the wavelet packet domain, associated with multimodal Markovian modeling adapted for the analysis of lung sounds (high intra and interpatient variability, low signal to noise ratio SNR) (*http://lsiit-miv.u-strasbg.fr/lsiit/perso/collet/*) [21,22]. Innovative vagueness (fuzzy) and uncertainty (probability) concepts on the observed data were developed and implemented successfully and resulted in the defining of an early statistical marker of asthma. These studies also focused on the detection of crackles using a deconvolution method (Bernoulli Gaussian model) allowing the density of the crackles to be quantified [4].

It should be mentioned that, in collaboration with the team led by Professor A. Dieterlen (University of Haute Alsace, Mulhouse, France), our team at the University Hospital of Strasbourg are also trialing a complementary approach in the field of cardiac signal analysis (PRI project [*see above*]).

Ultimately, there is scope for these different innovations to be combined in the future after refining and re-valuation of the procedures involved (using strict protocols similar to those used for drug development), to create new "communicating," "intelligent" stethoscopes.

6. Advances and innovations in the realm of the stethoscope

Today's technology, along with developments in modern medicine means that in the near future a communicating, wireless stethoscope will soon become available. This stethoscope will enable the recording, automated analysis and visualization of auscultatory signals [6,9].

INFRAL, a company (with whom we collaborate) based in Strasbourg, France, has developed several prototypes, with the aim of creating an intelligent communicating stethoscope system, which combines a diagnostic aid with tools for visualization and automated analysis [4].

This diagnostic aid is not only a helpful tool which assists physicians in making rapid decisions, but it will also allow developments in the field of telemedicine, for example; by the establishment of a database of auscultation sounds, by enabling the exchange of sounds between physicians and by allowing auscultation to be performed "from a distance" e.g. when seeking further expertise, etc. More importantly, it will allow auscultation to enter the field of fact-based medicine [6,9].

Figure 8 depicts one of the intelligent stethoscope prototypes, which uses *Bluetooth* to communicate with a PC, hand held computer or smartphone. This prototype was developed initially in the ASAP project (input of ALCATEL LUCENT), than by INFRAL, combining our expertise from several research projects as well as in the field of human sounds analysis, electronic stethoscope, e-health, e-teaching [4].

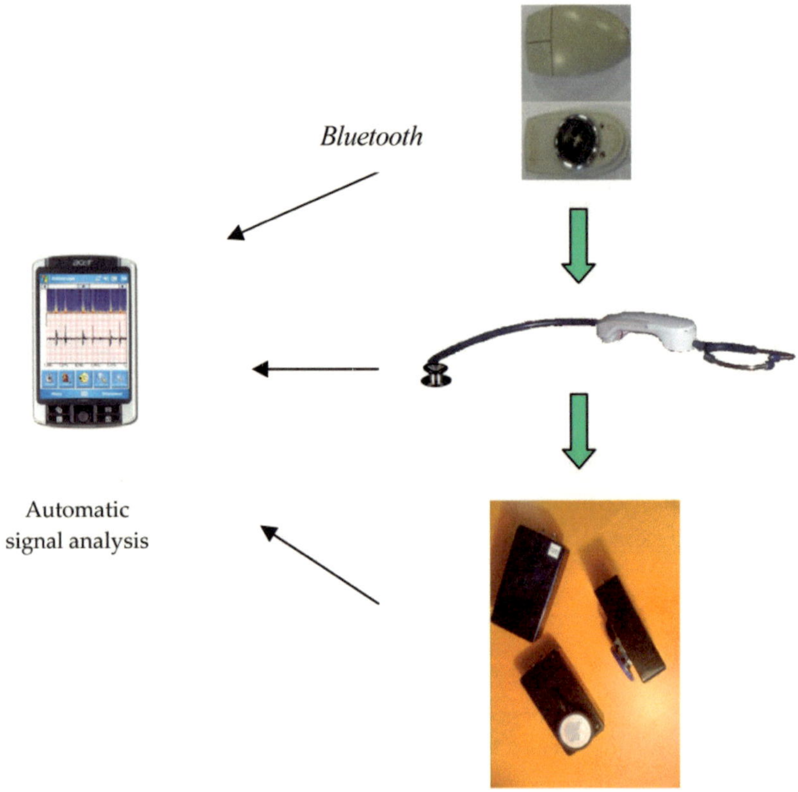

Figure 8. Several prototypes of intelligent (automatic signal analysis) communicating (Bluetooth) stethoscope system developed by our team in Strasbourg, France in different research projects, in collaboration mainly with LANNEXT, ALCATEL LUCENT, and currently with INFRAL [4].

In practical terms, a certain number of modern stethoscope models already feature functions for recording, storing and transmitting sounds. **Table 3** presents an overview of the major "electronic" stethoscope models currently available on the market and those, which we have tested [4,23]. The following section outlines two examples of new intelligent communicating stethoscope systems that we tested in clinical practice in our Department.

	Frequency bands and implemented filters	Communication mode	Additional Information	Ref	Price
Andromed	Presence of filers (high-pass at 200 Hz)	Wired connection		[Andromed 08a] [Andromed 08b]	
Jabes	Diaphragm mode (lung): 200 to 500 Hz Bell mode (heart) : 20 to 200 Hz Wide mode : 20 to 1000 Hz	Wired connection		[Jabes 08]	$299- $389
Stethoflux			Coupling of acoustic stethoscope and integrated continuous wave doppler	[Stethoflux 08]	$960
Welch-Allyn	20 - 20000 Hertz ; although two modes are present : the bell mode (heart) 20-420 Hz, and the diaphragm mode (lungs) 350-1900 Hz	Wired connection	Integrated ECG	[WelchAllyn 08]	$225 - $240
3M Littmann	Bell mode (20-200 Hz), diaphragm mode (100-500 Hz) and extended mode (20-1000 Hz).	Infrared	Transfer and display of sounds require additional time and investment by the physician conducting the auscultation Differed viewing and not in real time	[Littmann 08]	$465 - $674 (4100WS model)
Thinklabs	Filter for adjusting sound in bell/diaphragm mode, and acoustic mode.		Analysis software derived from Audacity	[Thinklabs 08]	$400 - $500
Cardionics	8 filters enabling the attenuation or amplification of 8 different frequency bands	Wired (jack)	Also has a complement system enabling ECG capability	[Cardionics O8a][Cardionics O8b]	$335 - $575

	Frequency bands and implemented filters	Communication mode	Additional Information	Ref	Price
Cardionics – Stethographics	8 filters enabling the attenuation or amplification of 8 different frequency bands	Wire (jack)	Multi probes	[Stethographics 08]	$279 - $489

Table 3. Principal characteristics of electronic stethoscopes currently available commercially [**4**].

The JABES *Life Sound System* is an auscultatory system composed of the JABES *Electronic Stethoscope* and JABES *Life Sound Analyzer* software. JABES hold the patent to this stethoscope technology, which consists primarily of an analog amplifier that can amplify body sounds up to 20 times. Hand tremor and ambient noise is minimized using information provided by the manufacturer, but in reality noise from the chest piece is very important.

The stethoscope offers various modes of auscultation: *Bell, Diaphragm* or *Wide*, each with 7 levels of volume control. Auscultation modes are reported to imitate the behavior of an acoustic stethoscope. Moreover, the system includes filters that reject certain frequency ranges in order to focus on lung or heart signals.

The JABES *Life Sound System* software allows the physician to record the body sounds of the patient directly onto his PC in order to view the phonocardiogram. In addition, heart and lungs sounds as well as the heartbeat can be visualized in real time.

The connection between the stethoscope and the PC or external recording equipment comprises a cable connected to the PC or external recorder jack socket. Sounds can be recorded on the PC in MP3 format, but are not documented. In particular, the sample sounds are not accompanied by tags (i.e. basic information such as the area over which the sample was taken).

It is also significant that sounds cannot be transmitted in "real-time" – hence simultaneous auscultation from a distance is not possible: the signal must first be recorded on the PC, before it can be transferred via email, CD or USB flash drive (for a second opinion). Thus because of these limitations, in our opinion it is not suitable for teaching purposes.

The 3M™ LITTMANN stethoscope (LITTMANN 08) is an electronic stethoscope that allows to 6 different sound recordings during auscultation. The sounds are stored directly in .wav format in the internal memory of the stethoscope.

The practitioner can then, through an analog connection to the PC (i.e. external microphone jack), or via an infrared link, transfer the sounds onto his PC for viewing using specific software provided by 3M.

This stethoscope allows sound to be amplified up to 18 times. It has several features including: ambient mechanical noise reduction technology, configurable filters with 3 frequency response modes for listening to the heart, lungs and other human body sounds: bell mode (20-200 Hz), diaphragm mode (100-500 Hz) and extended mode (20-1000 Hz).

The features are very similar to those of the JABES stethoscope; however this system is much more expensive. The stethoscope allows the physician to view the auscultatory sounds; although the display image is delayed and not in real time. Moreover, the transfer of sounds and their display require both additional cost and time. During auscultation it is not possible to visualize how the frequency spectrum of the signal changes with time, making the examination unsystematic, complicated, and invariably much longer.

It should be noted that the electronic stethoscopes currently on the market all have analog amplifiers, providing the option of connecting to a PC through the analog microphone jack socket [4]. In order to simulate "defects" introduced by acoustic stethoscopes, these electronic stethoscopes all offer analog filters that supposedly mimic the behavior of the bell or chest piece of the acoustic stethoscope. Finally, the wired connection between the stethoscope and the storage/processing device (PC or hand held computer or smartphone) is a major handicap in terms of user ergonomics.

7. Perspectives for the use of the new intelligent communicating stethoscope system in telemedicine in the field of chronic pathologies

Moreover, applications, including diagnosis establishment, monitoring and data exchange through Internet are obviously complementary tools to objective and automatic auscultation sounds analysis. Sensors devices will allow long duration monitoring for patient at home or at hospital. It could also be a useful solution for less-developed countries and remote communities... In addition, this type of system has the great advantage to keep the non-invasive and less expensive characteristics of auscultation.

The European based project, known as E-PERION, aims to develop telemedicine by using a platform which enables "secure" home support for fragile patients and/or those with chronic diseases (LEAD-ERA tender, 2010) (**Figure 9**). An intelligent communicating stethoscope system is one the deployed devices, especially in patients with respiratory and/or cardiac failure. This project is developped by INFRAL company (based in Strasbourg, France), in association with our team in Strasbourg.

This company is actively involved in the design and manufacture of modular and portable devices, which enable the transfer of essential medical data (*http://infral-systems.com/*). Such devices use innovative concepts to register and transmit vital parameters from medical devices.

In clinical practice, the most interesting and immediate advantages offered by this tool include:

- the ability to strengthen clinical evidence in favor of a particular diagnosis by visualization of the acoustic "pattern" of the sound;
- the ability to monitor the evolution of a pathology, by recording findings in a given individual;
- and the ability to share data, allowing the exchange of data between health care professionals (using an infrastructure similar to that of the ASAP project)).

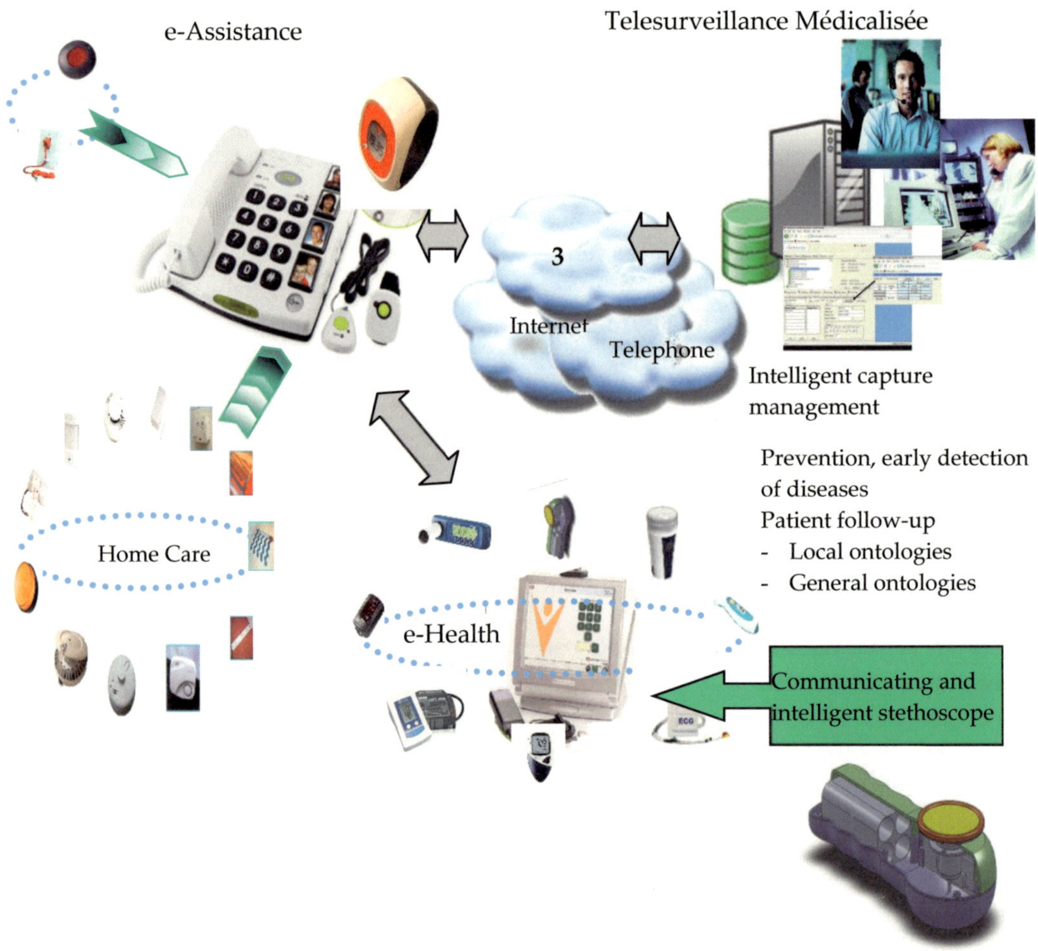

Figure 9. Prototype of a telemedicine platform enabling the "secure" home support of frail subjects and patients with chronic diseases, and integrating a “communicating” and “intelligent” stethoscope (*with the permission of INFRAL Company*).

8. Conclusions

Conventional auscultation is subjective and not easily shared. Modern medical technology allows us to optimize ausculatory findings and hence achieve a correct diagnosis by physically characterizing sounds through recordings, visualization and automated analysis systems. The development and availability of novel tools based on innovations in science and communications technology provide the clinician with an invaluable aid in order to achieve an early objective diagnosis, as well as offering increased sensitivity and reproducibility of auscultatory findings. Such advances have not only led to the development and use of new intelligent communicating stethoscope systems, but they have also significantly contributed to the revival of telemedicine, particularly as a diagnostic and teaching aid, e-teachnig and pedagogy.

Author details

Emmanuel Andrès
Department of Internal Medicine B, University Hospital of Strasbourg (HUS), Strasbourg, France
Unit of Human Sounds Analysis, University of Medicine, University of Strasbourg (UdS), Strasbourg, France
Laboratory of Research in Pedagogy in Human Health University of Strasbourg, Strasbourg, France

9. References

[1] Morton E. Tavel has given a good review on cardiac auscultation in the paper of "Cardiac Auscultation: A Glorious Past--And It Does Have a Future!". *Circulation* 2006; 113:1255-59.

[2] Reichert S, Gass R, Andrès E. Analyse des sons auscultatoires pulmonaires. *ITBM-RBM* 2007; 28: 169-80.

[3] Sovijarvi. A, Dalmasso, F. Vanderschoot J *et al.* Definition of terms for applications of respiratory sounds. *Eur Respir Rev* 2000; 77: 597-610.

[4] Andrès E, Hajjam A. Advances and innovations in the field of auscultation. *Health Technol* 2012; 2: 5-16.

[5] Andrès E, Reichert S, Gass R, Brandt C. A French national research project to the creation of an auscultation's school: the ASAP project. *Eur J Intern Med* 2009; 20: 323-7.

[6] Andrès E, Brandt C, Gass R. De l'intérêt de caractériser les sons de l'auscultation pulmonaire à la création d'une école de l'auscultation… *Presse Med* 2008; 37: 925-7.

[7] Sovijarvi AR, Malmberg LP, Charbonneau G, Vandershoot J. Characteristics of breath sounds and adventitious respiratory sounds. *Eur Respir Rev* 2000; 10: 591–6.

[8] Sovijarvi A, Vanderschoot J, Earis JE. Standardization of computerised respiratory sound analysis. *Eur Respir Rev* 2000; 10: 585-91.

[9] Andrès E, Brandt C, Gass R, Reichert S. Nouveaux développements dans le domaine de l'auscultation. *Rev Pneumol Clin* 2010; 66: 209-13.

[10] Elphick HE, Ritson S, Rodgers H, Everard ML. When a wheeze is not a wheeze: acoustic analysis of breath sounds in infants. *Eur Respir J* 2000; 16: 593-7.

[11] Kompis M, Pasterkamp H, Wodicka GR. Acoustic imaging of the human chest. *Chest* 2001; 120: 1309-21.

[12] Sestini P, Renzoni E, Rossi M, Beltrami V, Vagliasindi M. Multimedia presentation of lung sounds as learning aid for medical students. *Eur Respir J* 1995; 8: 783-8.

[13] Andrès E, Brandt C, Mecili M, Meyer N. Intérêt d'une démarche pédagogique structurée associée à de nouveaux outils de visualisation des signaux auscultatoires dans le cadre de l'apprentissage de la sémiologie auscultatoire: Étude prospective auprès de 30 étudiants du deuxième cycle des études médicales. *Pédagogie Med* 2012: *in press*.

[14] Myint WW, Dillard B. An electronic stethoscope with diagnosis capability. *Southeastern Symposium on System Theory. Proceedings of the 33rd*, pp. 133-137, 2001.

[15] Charbonneau G, Ademovic E, Cheetham B, Malmberg LP. Basic techniques for respiratory sound analysis. *Eur Respir Rev* 2000; 10: 625-35.

[16] Earis JE, Cheetham B. Current method used for computerised respiratory sound analysis. *Eur Respir Rev* 2000; 10: 586-90.

[17] Reichert S, Gass R, Kehayoff Y, Brandt C, Andrès E. Analysis of respiratory sounds: state of the art. *Clinical Medicine Circulatory Respiratory Pulmonary Medicine* 2008; 2: 45-58.

[18] Earis JE, Cheetham BM. Future perspectives for respiratory sound research. Techniques for respiratory sound analysis. *Eur Respir Rev* 2000; 10: 636–640.

[19] Cheetham B, Charbonneau G, Giordano A, Helisto P, Vanderschoot J. Digitization of data for respiratory sound recordings. *Eur Respir Rev* 2000; 10: 621-4.

[20] Vannuccini L, Earis JE, Helistö P *et al.* Capturing and preprocessing of respiratory sounds. *Eur Respir Rev* 2000; 10: 616-20.

[21] Le Cam S, Salzenstein F, Collet C. Fuzzy pairwise Markov chain to segment correlated noisy data. *Signal Processing* 2008; 88: 2526–41.

[22] Salzenstein F, Collet C, Le Cam S, Hatt M. Non-stationary fuzzy Markov chain. *Pattern Recognition Letters* 2007; 28: 2201–08.

[23] Hung K., Luk BL, Choy WH, Tsa BI, Tso SK. Multifunction stethoscope for telemedicine. *Medical Devices and Biosensors. 2nd IEEE/EMBS International Summer School* on, pp. 87-89, 2004.

Chapter 7

Phonocardiogram Signal Processing Module for Auto-Diagnosis and Telemedicine Applications

Ali Moukadem, Alain Dieterlen and Christian Brandt

Additional information is available at the end of the chapter

http://dx.doi.org/10.5772/48447

1. Introduction

The advancement of technology has paved the way for signal processing methods to be implemented and applied in many simple tools useful in everyday life. This is most notable in the medical technology field where contributions involving the intelligent applications have boosted the quality of diagnosis. Proposing an objective signal processing methods able to extract relevant information from biosignals is a great challenge in telemedicine and auto-diagnosis fields.

For the cardiac system, many signals can be treated and monitored; ElectroCardioGram (ECG), PhonoCardioGram (PCG), Echo/Doppler and pressure monitor, see Figure 1.

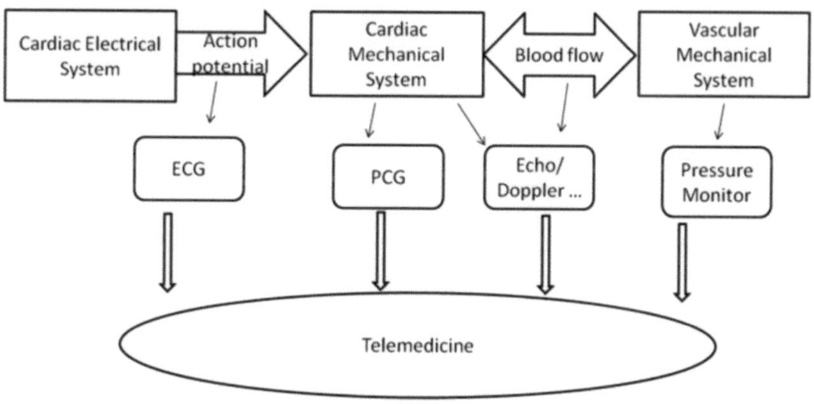

Figure 1. The cardiac activity with different measurable signals [1].

The interest of this book chapter is the PCG signal. PCG and auscultation are noninvasive, low-cost and accurate for diagnosing some heart diseases.

The PCG signal confirms, and mostly, refines the auscultation data and provides further information about the acoustic activity concerning the chronology of the pathological signs in the cardiac cycle, by locating them with respect to the normal heart sounds. The cardiac sounds are by definition non-stationary signals, and are located within the low frequency range, approximately between 10 and 750 Hz.

The analysis of the cardiac sounds, solely based on the human ear, remains insufficient for a reliable diagnosis of cardiac pathologies, and for a clinician to obtain all the qualitative and quantitative information about cardiac activity especially in the field of time intervals.

Information, such as the temporal localization of the heart sounds, the number of their internal components, their frequency content, and the significance of diastolic and systolic murmurs, could all be studied directly on the PCG signal. In order to recognize and classify cardiovascular pathologies, advanced methods and techniques of signal processing and artificial intelligence will be used.

For that, different approaches could be considered for improve the electronic stethoscope:

Tool with embedded autonomous analysis, simple for home use by the general public for the purpose of auto-diagnosis, monitoring and warning in case of necessity.

Tool with sophisticated analysis (coupled to a PC, Bluetooth link) for the use of professionals in order to make an in-depth medical diagnosis and to train the medical students.

Whatever the approach, one of the first and most important phases in the analysis of heart sounds, is the segmentation of heart sounds. Heart sound segmentation partitions the PCG signals into cardiac cycles and further into S1 (first heart sound), systole, S2 (second heart sound) and diastole.

Identification of the two phases of the cardiac cycle and of the heart sounds with robust differentiation between S1 and S2 even in the presence of additional heart sounds and/or murmurs is a first step in this challenge. Then there is a need to measure accurately S1 and S2 allowing the progression to automatic diagnosis of heart murmurs with the distinction of ejection and regurgitation murmurs.

This phase of autonomous detection, without the help of ECG is based on signal processing tools such as: Shannon energy [2], Hilbert Transform [3], high order statistics [1], hidden Markov model [4] …

In this chapter we present a new module for heart sounds segmentation based on time-frequency analysis (S-Transform). The goal of this study is to develop a generic tool, suitable for clinical and home monitoring use, robust to noise, and applicable to diverse pathological and normal heart sound signals without the necessity of any previous information about the subject. The proposed segmentation module can be divided into three main blocks: localization of heart sounds, boundaries detection of the localized heart sounds and classification block to distinguish between S1 and S2.

The proposed methods are evaluated based on a database of 80 subjects (40 pathologic). This study is made under the control of an experienced cardiologist, in with the aim of validating the results of each method.

This chapter is organized as follows: Section 2 describes the data base used in this study. It is followed by the Section 3 which describes the different methods proposed for the segmentation module (localization, boundaries detection and classification). The results and discussion are presented in Section 4 and Sections 5 and 6 give the future research and the conclusion.

2. Data base

Several factors affect the quality of the acquired signal, above all, the type of the electronic stethoscope, its mode of use, the patient's position during auscultation, and the surrounding noise. According to the cardiologist's experience, it's preferable that the signals remain unrefined; filtration will only be applied subsequently in the purpose of signal analysis. For this reason we used prototype stethoscopes produced by Infral Corporation, and comprising an acoustic chamber in which a sound sensor is inserted. Electronics of signal conditioning and amplification are inserted in a case along with a Bluetooth standard communication module.

Different cardiologists equipped with a prototype electronic stethoscope have contributed to a campaign of measurements in the Hospital of Strasbourg. In parallel, 2 prototypes have dedicated to the MARS500 project promoted by ESA, in order to collect signals form 6 volunteers (astronauts). The use of prototype electronic stethoscopes by different cardiologists makes the database rich in terms of qualitative diversity of collected sounds, which in turn makes the heart sounds localization more realistic.

The sounds are recorded with 16 bits accuracy and 8000Hz sampling frequency in a wave format, using the software "Stetho" developed under Alcatel-Lucent license.

The dataset contains 80 subjects, including 40 cardiac pathologies sounds which contain different systolic murmurs. Each subject corresponds to one recording sound. The length of each sound is 8 seconds.

3. Method

3.1. Preprocessing

At first the original signal is decimated by factor 4 from 8000 Hz to 2000 Hz sampling frequency and then the signal is filtered by a high-pass filter with cut-off frequency of 30 Hz, to eliminate the noise collected by the prototype stethoscope. The filtered signal is refiltered reverse direction so that there is no time delay in the resulting signal. Then, the Normalization is applied by setting the variance of the signal to a value of 1. The resulting signal is expressed by:

$$x_{norm}(t) = \frac{x(t)}{|\max(x(t))|} \quad (1)$$

3.2. Localization of heart sounds

The localization algorithms operating on PCG data try to emphasize heart sound occurrences with an initial transformation that can be classified into three main categories: frequency based transformation, morphological transformations and complexity based transformations [1]. The transformation try to maximize the distance between the heart sounds and the background noise, and the result is smoothed and tresholded in order to apply a peak detector algorithm. We note here, that the main goal of heart sound localization is to locate the first and the second heart sounds but without distinguishing the two from each other and without detecting the boundaries of located sounds.

3.3. SRBF localization method

We proposed the RBF method as a transformation to emphasize heart sounds and it was shown to have a good performance on low level noise signals [5]. However, In the presence of high level of noise, the performance of the RBF method decreases. This was not surprising because the method operates directly on the heart sound without any feature extraction step. To deal with this problem, we proposed a method for heart sounds localization named SRBF [6]. This method aims at extracting the envelope of the signal by applying the features extracted from the S-Transform matrix of the heart sound signal to the radial basis function (RBF) neural network. Compared with other existing methods for heart sounds localization, SRBF was shown to have a significant enhancement in term of sensitivity and positive predictive value and the robustness of this method was shown against additive white Gaussian noise.

We will briefly explain the different steps of the SRBF method:

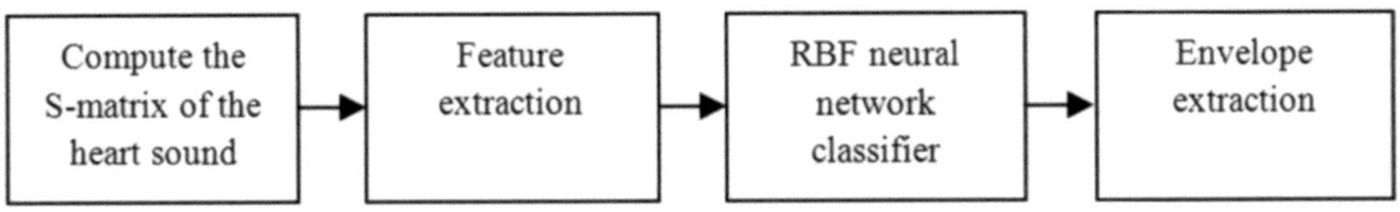

Figure 2. Block Diagram of SRBF Method

1. The S-Transform of the heart sound is calculated. A frequency range of 0-100 Hz was used to cover the main frequency band of S1 and S2 and to avoid murmurs which have in general a spectral energy above the frequency of 100 Hz [7].
2. A sliding window of 50 ms (so 100 samples) was operated on the S-matrix and an overlap of 75% was chosen. The feature extraction is done by applying some standard statistical techniques and transformations like Root Mean Square (RMS), the maximum and the average of each column of the S-matrix. Each array (100 samples) was divided into 5 segments and the mean of calculated features of each segment was calculated and

taken as input to the classifier. So for each step we have a 100 by 100 matrix which gives 15 descriptors.

3. A RBF neural network classifier is used and trained on two heart sounds samples (S1 and S2) and two no heart sound samples (systole, diastole) selected randomly from the database. The target is fixed to 1 for S1 or S2 and 0 for the other components. So the envelope of the signal is constructed by the output of the RBF neural network.

3.4. SSE localization method

A new method for the localization of heart sounds is proposed in this study (SSE). It uses the S-matrix like the SRBF method (0-100 Hz) and it calculates the Shannon Energy (SE) of the local spectrum calculated by the S-transform for each sample of the signal *x(t)*. Then, the extracted envelope is smoothed by applying an average filter (Figure 3).

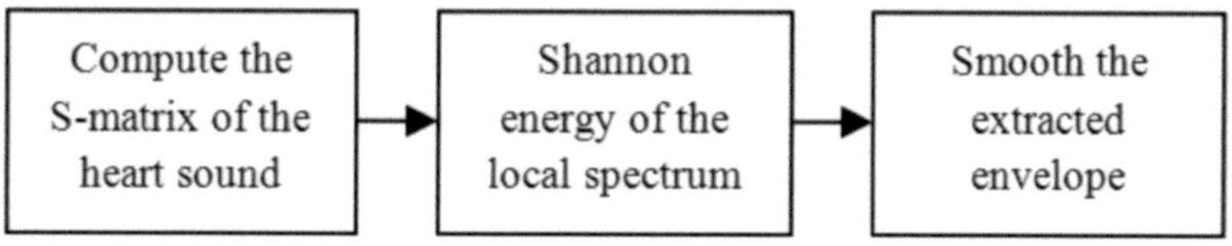

Figure 3. Block Diagram of SSE Method

The S-Transform proposed in [8], of a time series x(t) is:

$$S(\tau,f)=\int_{-\infty}^{\infty} x(t)w(\tau-t)e^{-2\pi ift}dt \tag{2}$$

Where the window function *w(τ-t)* is chosen as:

$$w(t,f)=\frac{1}{\sigma(f)\sqrt{2\pi}}e^{\frac{-t}{2\sigma f^2}} \tag{3}$$

And *σ(f)* is a function of frequency as:

$$\sigma(f)=\frac{1}{|f|} \tag{4}$$

The proposed SSE method calculates the Shannon energy of each column of the extracted S-matrix as follows:

$$SSE(x_i)=\sum_{j=0}^{n} S(j,i)^2\log(S(j,i)^2) \tag{5}$$

Each column of the S-matrix represents the local frequency at a specific sample. The advantage of the Shannon energy transformation is its capacity to emphasize the medium intensities and to attenuate low intensities of the signal which represents the local spectrum in the case the

SSE method. The main difference between the SSE and the SRBF method is the training phase needed for the RBF module. The RBF neural network in the SRBF method can be considered as a non-linear filter which is replaced with a simple average filter in the SSE method.

3.5. Boundaries detection algorithm: An optimized S-transform approach

The boundaries detection algorithm aims at estimating the onset and the endpoint of the located heart sounds. Accurate boundaries estimation is a very important step in the heart sound segmentation module and it is essential for the extraction of meaningful features from each part of heart cycles in order to perform an auto-diagnosis process.

3.5.1. Overview of existing methods

Different boundaries detection algorithms exists in the literature, in [2] the boundaries are estimated by applying a threshold on the extracted envelope of the signal, this is not be accurate for some cardiac cycles, because the envelope threshold level is used based on the average value of the whole recordings periods. The same authors propose another algorithm that employs the STFT (Short Time Fourier Transform) to explore the time-frequency domain of the signal [9]. Authors quantify the spectrogram at each segment to two values by applying a threshold that reserves 60% of the signal energy, however, it is not clear how the energy of the signal is calculated and the accuracy of the algorithm is not mentioned. In [10] authors use some biomedical features of heart sounds (S1 and S2) like the maximum duration of S1 and S2 to determine the limit of estimated boundaries, the disadvantage of this method is that the estimation of energy of the signal is based on the time domain only, so in the presence of high level of noise the performance of this method will decrease dramatically.

3.5.2. The OSSE algorithm

In this chapter, we propose a new algorithm to estimate the heart sounds boundaries. The proposed algorithm tries to optimize the energy concentration of the S-transform at each located sound by using a window width optimization method. The envelope of the optimized S-transform is then recalculated by using the SSE approach and an adaptive threshold is applied to determine the onset and the ending of each located heart sound. Let us assume that L is the time located sounds after applying the localization method on the heart sound and $S(M,N)$ is the S-matrix of the heart sound where M represents the frequency domain and N the time domain.

The block diagram of the proposed algorithm (OSSE) is shown below (Figure 4).

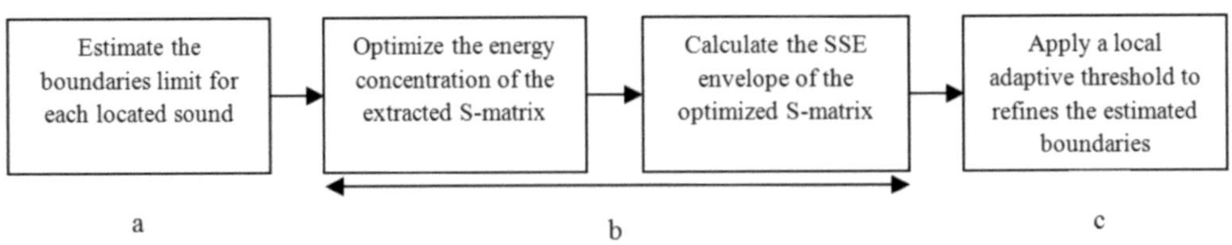

Figure 4. The block diagram of the OSSE Method

a. Estimate the boundaries limit

The boundaries limits are estimated basing on the fact that the maximum duration of S1 and S2 is 150 ms [11]. So a 150ms window is applied in the proximity of detected S1 and S2 peaks which covers 75ms in the backward direction of the *S*1 or *S*2 peak and 75ms in the forward direction.

b. Optimized S-transform

Many studies tried to improve the TF representation of the S-transform[12-14]. The main study in the literature interested to optimize the energy concentration in the TF domain was in [14]. That is, to minimize the spread of the energy beyond the actual signal components. As it well known, the ideal time-frequency transformation should only be distributed along frequencies for the duration of signal components. So the neighboring frequencies would not contain any energy and the energy contribution of each component would not exceed its duration [15].

The energy concentration in the Time-Frequency (TF) domain is a very important parameter for the algorithms that aim to detect the duration of any given events in a signal. Therefore, it should hold the same importance for the boundaries detection algorithm of heart sounds based on time-frequency features. However, in some cases, the S-transform suffers from poor energy concentration in TF domain. Hence, the importance of an energy concentration optimization process to improve the boundaries estimation of the heart sounds.

The main approach is to optimize the width of the window used in the S-transform. The width of the Gaussian window can be controlled by several ways by adding a new parameter to the window equation. We use in this study the parameter p introduced in [14] and we investigate another parameter named α (see equation 6). Both of them control the Gaussian window width:

$$\sigma(f) = \frac{\alpha}{|f|^p} \tag{6}$$

We note here that in this study when α vary, p is fixed to 1, and when p vary, α is fixed to 1. The optimal value can be calculated in two methods; the first method calculates one global parameter, which is recommended for signals with constant or very slowly varying frequency components. The second method calculates the time-varying parameter which is more suitable for signals with fast varying frequency components. The disadvantage of the second approach is its high computational complexity which makes it unsuitable for applications where time is an important factor.

Based on the first approach, the optimization algorithm is applied on both parameters p and α, separately. The performance measure against each parameter is compared in section (5.2). The performance measure is based on the concentration measure (CM) proposed in [16]. For each α (or p) from a given set, the CM (α) can be expressed by [14]:

$$CM(\alpha) = \frac{1}{\int_{-\infty}^{+\infty}\int_{-\infty}^{+\infty} \left|S_x^{\alpha}(t,f)\right| dt df} \tag{7}$$

With $\overline{S_x^\alpha(t,f)}$ is the normalized energy of the S-transform for each α; it's given by:

$$\overline{S_x^\alpha(t,f)} = \frac{S_x^\alpha(t,f)}{\sqrt{\int_{-\infty}^{+\infty}\int_{-\infty}^{+\infty}\left|S_x^\alpha(t,f)\right|^2 dtdf}} \tag{8}$$

The CM (α) and CM (p) are calculated and compared for all existing S1 and S2 sounds in the database. We note again that the main objective is to enhance the concentration energy of the S-transform in order to detect precisely the boundaries of the located heart sounds. We consider the parameter that reaches a higher CM to be more appropriate for the heart sound signals.

c. The Adaptive threshold

Performing an optimized S-transform before calculating the SSE envelope makes the choice of threshold less sensitive to the variation of different heart sounds. In this study, a threshold which equals 10 % of the maximum value of the SSE envelope is applied to refine the estimated boundaries.

3.6. Distinguishing S1 and S2

Most of the existing methods for the segmentation of heart sounds use the feature of systole and diastole duration to classify the first heart sound (S1) and the second heart sound (S2) [1,17-18]. These time intervals can become problematic and useless in several clinical real life settings which are particularly represented by severe tachycardia or in tachyarrhythmia (Figure 5).

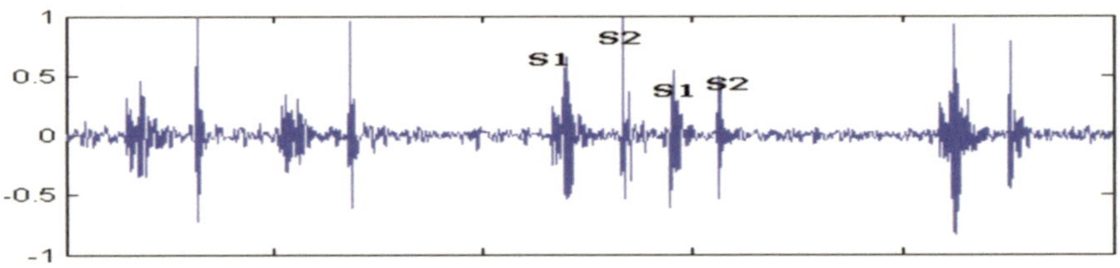

Figure 5. Example of an arrhythmic subject.

Consequently with the objective of development of a robust generic module for heart sound segmentation, we present in this chapter two feature extraction methods based on the Singular Value Decomposition (SVD) technique applied on the S-matrix, to classify S1 and S2. We investigate also, the ability of a new individual features based on the width of the optimized Gaussian window of the S-Transform, to discriminate between S1 and S2.

3.6.1. Feature extraction based on the S-Transform

The SVD is a powerful tool that provides a compact matrix or compact significant information about single signal. Different ways exist in the literature aims to represent the time-frequency matrix in a compact manner by using the SVD technique. In [19] authors extracted the eigenvalues of the time-frequency matrix. In [20] authors extended the method to also incorporate information from the eigenvectors to classify EEG seizures. In [21] the last technique is applied on the S-matrix in the aim to extract features for systolic heart murmur classification. Following this approach, this study proposes a feature extraction method for S1 and S2 classification.

The time-frequency analysis is performed by the S-Transform. The S-matrix Si of the extracted heart sound Hi is decomposed by the SVD technique as follows:

$$S_i = UDV^T \tag{9}$$

Where $U(M{\times}M)$ and $V(N{\times}N)$ are orthonormal matrices so their squared elements can be considered as density function[20], and $D(M{\times}N)$ is a diagonal matrix of singular values. The columns of the orthonormal matrices U and V are called the left and right eigenvectors which contains in this case the time and frequency domain information, respectively. The eigenvectors related to the largest singular values contain more information about the structure of the signal.

Based on our experience, in this study, the first left eigenvector and the first right eigenvector that correspond to the largest singular values are used for the feature extraction process. The histogram (10 bins) for each related distribution function is calculated based on the density function. Five feature vectors obtained by this method are tested in the classification process; the eigentime histogram vector U_1 (T-Features), the eigenfrequency histogram vector V_1 (F-Features), the singular values vector D_1 (SV Features) and the time-frequency vector $U_1\&V_1$ (TF Features). All vectors have a length of 10 features except the time-frequency vector that has a length of 20.

3.6.2. Feature extraction using the EMD

In the last few years, the Empirical Mode Decomposition (EMD) has been applied in many fields one of which the biomedical signal analysis, like the emotion classification in natural speech [22], analysis of gastroesphageal information [23]. EMD has been applied to a simulated heart sounds in [24] authors show that EMD provides clear information about the components of S1 and S2 and their instantaneous frequency behaviour. In [25] authors presented a feature analysis approach of heart sound based on the improved Hilbert-Huang Transform, and applied the improved HHT by Hilbert spectrum analysis of various cases of heart sounds. In this study, a new feature extraction method based on EMD technique and Shannon energy is proposed for S1 and S2 classification.

As an alternative to the binomial TF transforms, EMD performs a multi-resolution analysis of non-stationary and nonlinear signals without the use of kernels or mother waveforms. To calculate the Intrinsic Mode Functions (IMFs), the local maxima and minima of extracted heart sound $H_i(t)$are calculated. They are interpolated by using the cubic spline curves which generates the upper and lower envelopes, respectively. Then the mean contour $m_1(t)$ is calculated, and the first component $h_1(t)$ is given as follows:

$$h_1(t) = H_i(t) - m_1(t) \tag{10}$$

Now, h_1 has to be refined by a sifting process. In the second sifting iteration we obtain:

$$h_{11}(t) = h_1(t) - m_{11}(t) \tag{11}$$

Where m_{11} is an average contour between the upper and lower envelopes of h_1. This operation is repeated k times until h_{1k} can be considered as zero-mean according to some stopping criterion (Rilling et al., 2003). The first intrinsic mode function $IMF_1(t)$ is given as:

$$IMF_1(t) = h_{1(k-1)}(t) - m_{1k}(t) \tag{12}$$

$IMF_1(t)$ should contain the finest scale or the shortest period component of the signal. The residue signal $r_1(t)$ is given by:

$$r_1(t) = H_i(t) - IMF_1(t) \tag{13}$$

Considering r_1 as a new signal the sifting process explained below is repeated to obtain the second $IMF_2(t)$. Similarly, a series of intrinsic mode functions are obtained and the final residue $r_n(t)$ is calculated. The stop criterion is when $r_n(t)$ becomes a monotonic function.

The initial signal $H_i(t)$ can be reconstructed as follows:

$$H_i(t) = \sum_{j=1}^{n} IMF_j(t) + r_n \tag{14}$$

For each IMF vector, the Shannon Energy is calculated as:

$$SE_i = -\sum_{k=1}^{N} IMF_i^2(k).\log(IMF_i^2(k)) \tag{15}$$

Where $i=1,\ldots,4$ and N is the number of samples of IMF_i the Shannon energy is smoothed by using a median filter, and the feature vector is obtained by applying the same SVD approach used in section 2.5.1 at each calculated *IMF* (Figure 6). For each extracted heart sound the first four *IMF* is calculated. The others *IMF* don't contain relevant information about S1 and S2. Five feature vectors obtained by this method are tested in the classification process; FV1 (that correspond to IMF1 signal), FV2, FV3, FV4 and FV (that correspond to the average of calculated FVs). The length of each vector is 10.

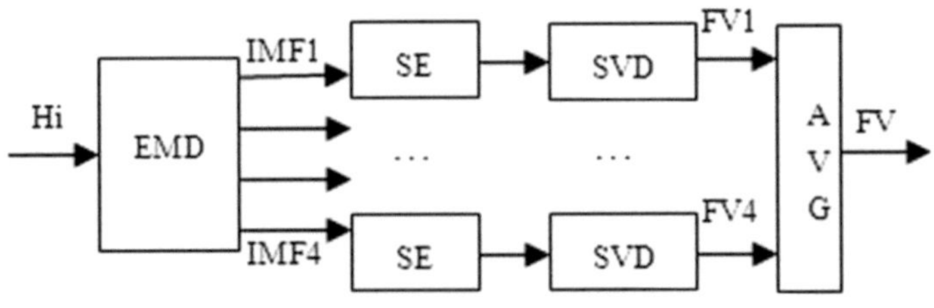

Figure 6. Feature vector (FV) of Heart Sounds (Hi) extracted using EMD and Shannon Energy (SE) before applying the SVD technique.

3.6.3. *New individual features*

The parameters α and p used to optimize the width of the Gaussian window of the S-Transform, are tested as a new individual features to discriminate between S1 and S2. It is known from a physiological point of view, that S1 is more complicated than S2 [26]. However, S2 in general contain higher frequency than S1. These physiological differences will necessarily lead to different time-frequency content behavior which we will aim to reveal with α and p parameters. Figure 7 shows a S1 and S2 signals examples with the corresponding optimized S-transform obtained with α=0.8 and 0.5, respectively.

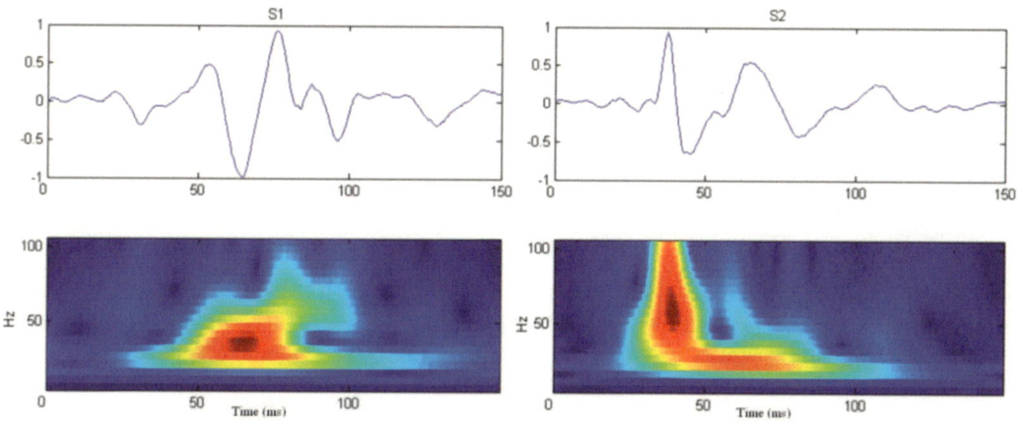

Figure 7. S1 and S2 signals (top), Optimized S-transform obtained with α=0.8 for S1 and α=0.5 for S2 (bottom).

4. Results and discussion

4.1. Localization methods

The performance of the SBRF and the SSE methods was measured as the methods capacity to locate S1 and S2 correctly. It was measured by sensitivity and positive predictive value:

$$Sensitivity = \frac{TP}{TP + FN} \tag{16}$$

And positive predictive value:

$$PPV = \frac{TP}{TP + FP} \tag{17}$$

A sound is true positive (TP) if it is correctly located, all others detected sounds are considered as false positive (FP) and all missed sounds are considered as false negative (FN).

Results in Table 1 show that SRBF method reaches a higher PPV (98%) than the SSE method for the clinical signals without any additive noise. However, SSE reaches a higher sensitivity

(96%) than the SRBF method (92%). The supervised approach performed by the RBF block in the SRBF method makes the extracted envelope more discriminative between the different parts of the signal than the unsupervised SSE method. Therefore, it is not surprising that the number of false detected sounds in the SRBF method is lower than the SSE method, which also explains the PPV results. The same reasons can also account for the false negative alarms which are higher in the SRBF method than the SSE method and which gives a higher sensitivity to the SSE method. In the presence of an additive white Gaussian noise, the performance of the SSE method is better with 93% sensitivity and 94% PPV. The robustness of both methods against noise is very significant. This is due to the advantage of performing a time-frequency analysis which makes methods more robust against noise. Figure 8 shows the envelopes extracted by the SSE and the SRBF method that correspond to a pathologic sound with a systolic murmur. Figure 9 shows the robustness of each method against white additive noise.

Method	Sensitivity	PPV	Sensitivity (Noise)	PPV (Noise)
SRBF	92%	98%	91%	93%
SSE	96%	95%	93%	94%

Table 1. Sensitivity and Positive Predictive Values for the SRBF and SSE methods applied on the clinical sounds set without and with additive Gaussian noise.

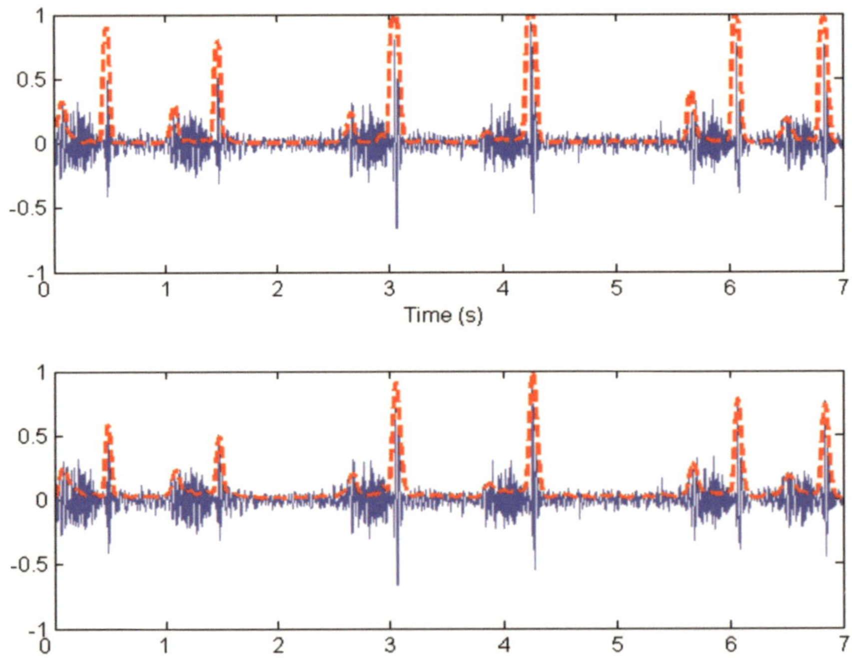

Figure 8. Envelope extraction (dashed lines) for a signal with systolic murmur, (top) SRBF envelope, (bottom) SSE envelope.

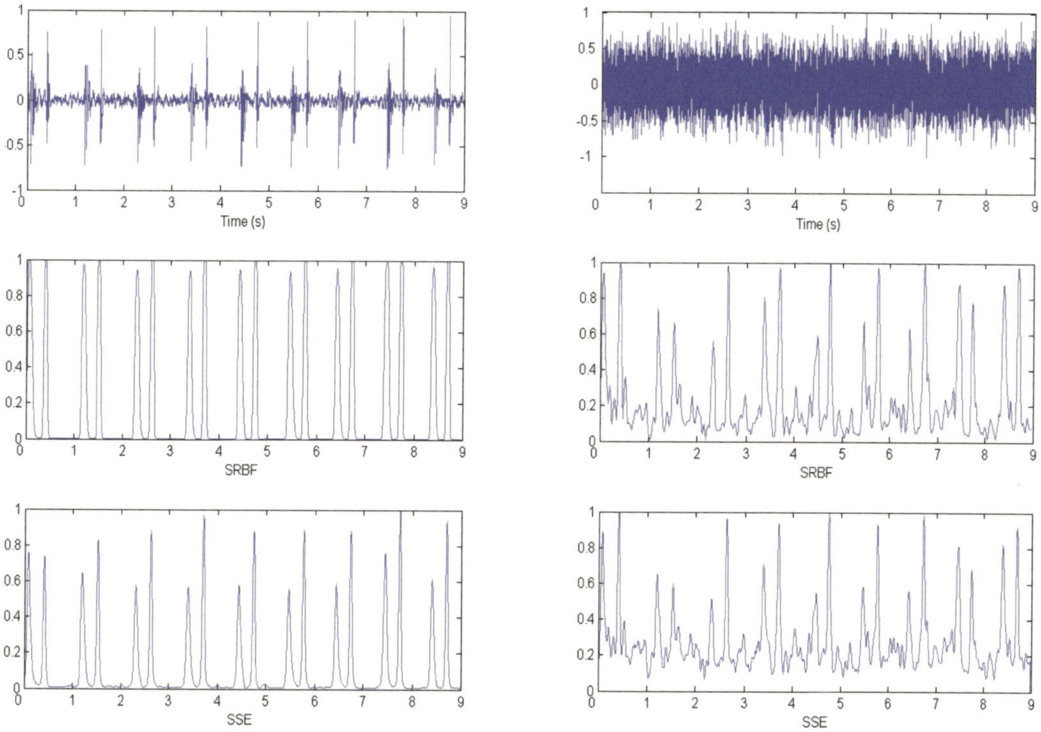

Figure 9. (top) Envelope extraction for two normal PCG signal without and with additive Gaussian noise, (middle) their SRBF envelopes, (bottom) their SSE envelopes.

4.2. Boundaries detection

The performance measure against each parameter is compared (Table2). The values of α and p are chosen from a set; $0 < \alpha < 2$, $0 < p < 2$, with a step of 0.1; so twenty values as total for each variable.

Heart Sounds	Optimal α	CM(α)	Optimal p	CM(p)	CM(α =1, p=1)
S1	0.82±0.45	0.0185±0.0017	1.1±0.5	0.0186±0.0018	0.0177±0.0015
S2	0.55±0.3	0.0186±0.0015	1.37±0.5	0.0186±0.0018	0.0175±0.0014
Total	0.68±0.37	0.0185±0.0016	1.23±0.5	0.0186±0.0018	0.0176±0.0015

Table 2. Performance measure given by the maximum values of CM (α) and CM (p) for a given parameters set of α and p, respectively.

The optimal α is reached when CM(α) is maximized, and the optimal p is reached when CM (p) is maximized. Results from Table 2 show that there are no significant differences between the two parameters α and p concerning the performance measure. However, results show an important difference between optimized concentration measure and standard concentration that correspond to the standard S-transform with α=1 and p=1. The maximum values of concentration measures CM (α) and CM (p), that corresponds to the optimum α

and p, respectively, are obtained with α <1 and p>1. This is can be explained by the fact that when α<1 and p>1, the Gaussian window of the S-transform is narrower (Figure 10), which improves the detection of the sudden changes in the signal, like the onset and the ending of the first and the second heart sounds. However, when a window is narrower in time domain, we loss in term of frequency resolution. The compromise is performed by the optimization process that operates on the variable that control the variance of the Gaussian window, α or p for example. The criterion of the performance is the concentration energy measure. The enhancement of energy concentration in the TF domain, influence clearly on the boundaries estimation results (Table 3).

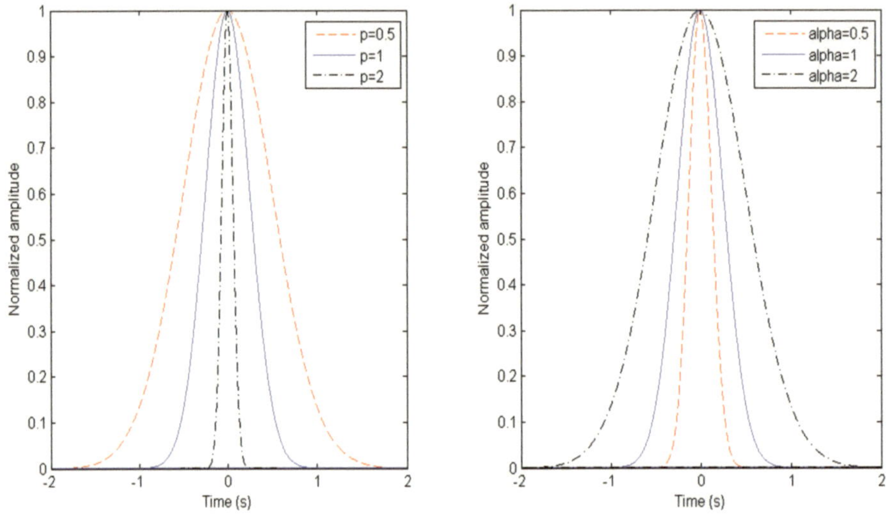

Figure 10. Normalized Gaussian window for different values of p (left) and for different values of α (right).

Method	S1(ms)	S1(Noise)	S2(ms)	S2 (Noise)
SSE	122.4±7.2	127.8±9.6	95.2±8.3	101.2±7.4
OSSE	110.7±4.32	113.6±6.5	69.1±5.4	77.9±8.2
Reference	105.8±6		74.8±5.65	

Table 3. S1 and S2 durations (ms) estimated by the SSE and OSSE methods with and without additive noise.

The "Reference" row in Table 3 represents the manual measures made by the cardiologists by using the software stetho developed under the license of Alcatel-Lucent. Results show the efficiency of optimizing the energy concentration of the S-transform in order to estimate more realistic boundaries for S1 and S2. Measures obtained by the SSE algorithm (without optimizing the S-transform) are always higher than the results given by the OSSE algorithm where an optimization process is performed. This is not surprising since the OSSE algorithm has a better energy concentration in the TF domain, which minimizes the spread of the energy beyond the S1 and the S2. Figure 11 shows the boundaries detection results, with and without optimization of the S-transform, applied on a S2 example and figure 12 shows the OSSE results applied on the entire heart sounds (normal and pathologic).

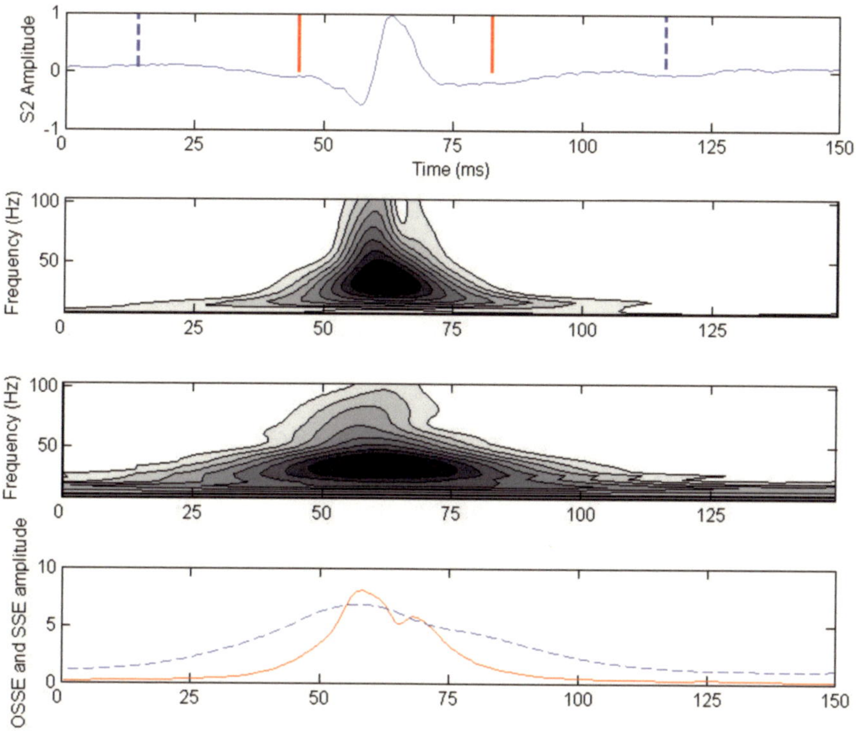

Figure 11. (top) S2 signal with two detected boundaries calculated by the optimized S-transform and the standard S-transform (dashed line), S-transform with the optimum value $\alpha=0.5$ ($p=1$), standard S-transform with $\alpha=1$ ($p=1$), (bottom) SSE envelope for the optimized S-transform and standard S-transform (dashed line).

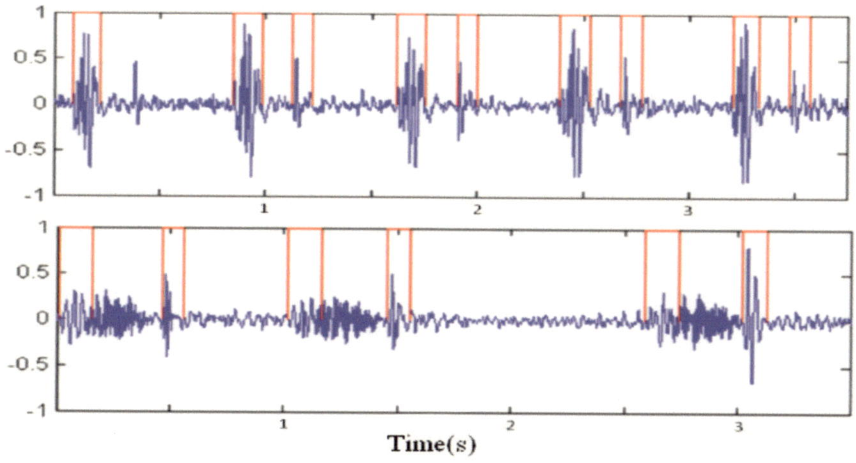

Figure 12. OSSE method applied on a normal heart sound (top) and pathological heart sound (bottom).

4.3. Feature extraction for S1 and S2 classification

4.3.1. Evaluating the feature vectors obtained by the SVD technique

The localization of heart sounds is established by using the SSE method. The boundaries of the heart sounds are determined by the OSSE algorithm. The results were visually inspected by a cardiologist and erroneously extracted heart sounds were excluded from the study. The feature extraction process extracts a feature vector per extracted sound S_i (S1 or S2) and each of these vectors is averaged across available extracted sounds from each subject. So from each subject in the database, we obtain one S1 feature vector and one S2 feature vector to use in the training and classification process.

A 3-Neirest Neighbor (KNN) classifier is used to evaluate the performance of the four feature vectors obtained by the two methods and the 5-fold approach is used for cross validation. The choice of KNN classifier was based on its simplicity of and its robustness to a noisy training data.

The time domain feature vector reaches 92% classification rate, however, the frequency feature vector reaches 85% classification rate (81% sensitivity and 88% specificity). The Time-Frequency vector (TF Features) reaches the higher classification rate with 95% sensitivity and 97% specificity. The singular values are almost indistinguishable from each other and it is shown by the low classification rate for the SV features. For the EMD based method, the FV feature vector reaches a high classification rate with 94% sensitivity and 97% specificity (Table4).

KNN	T-Features	F-Features	SV Features	TF Features	FV1	FV2	FV3	FV4	FV
Sensitivity	92%	81%	60%	95%	88%	81%	82%	65%	94%
Specificity	92%	88%	65%	97%	91%	97%	94%	95%	97%

Table 4. Sensitivity and specificity for the nine extracted feature vectors evaluated by a KNN classifier.

In most cases seen in the medical field, S2 has a higher frequency than S1. This is due to the fact that S2 is the heart sound associated with the closure of the aortic valve in a context of high left ventricular pressure, the mitral closing occurring at low left ventricular pressure (S1). However, this criterion cannot be generalized on all real life cases because some medical conditions are characterized by S2 frequency content lower than S1 frequency content. Hence, the importance of time-frequency and multi-resolution based features approach, especially in a generic module, which can explain the high performance obtained with the TF and FV features vectors.

4.3.2. Evaluating α and p to discriminate S1 and S2

The parameters used in the optimization process (section 3.3.2) to determine the boundaries of each extracted sound S_i (S1 or S2) are averaged across available extracted sounds from each subject. So from each subject in the database, we obtain one S1 feature (α or p) and one S2 feature (α or p).

The main objective is to investigate the ability of these features to discriminate between S1 and S2. The probability that the two groups (S1 and S2) comes from distributions with different medians is calculated for each feature (α and p) by the Mann-Whitney-U-test ($p<0.005$). The receiver Operating Characteristic Curve (ROC) is also calculated for each feature and the Areas under the ROC Curve (AUC) are showed in figure 13.

The Results are presented in Table 5. Significant differences between the groups, with 95% confidence are found for both features α and p.

Feature	p-value	AUC	Sensitivity	Specificity
α	<0.0001	0.83	0.79	0.72
p	0.0047	0.64	0.609	0.671

Table 5. Significant values (U-test), AUC values, sensitivity and specificity for the parameters α and p when used to distinguished between S1 and S2.

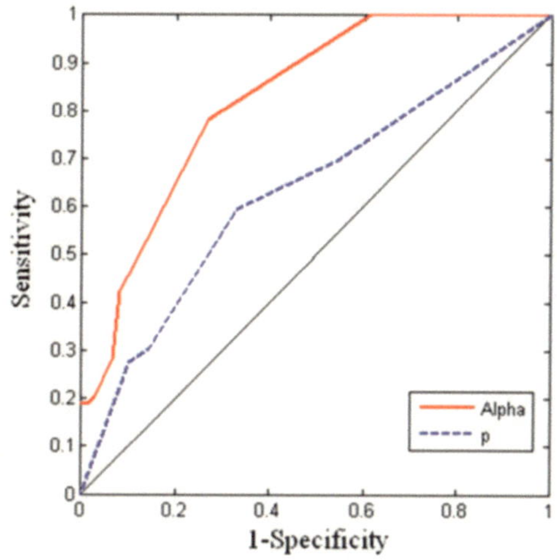

Figure 13. ROC curves for α and p parameters.

The classification results are promising for the parameter α (AUC =0.83). This is very interesting since this parameter was also used to refine the boundaries detection of S1 and S2. However, the results of the parameter p are significantly lower than the results of α (AUC =0.64). This gives a primary idea about the sensitivity of each parameter against the clinical signals. Further measures and tests should verify or deny this hypothesis.

5. Future research

5.1. Classification of heart sounds

A new time-frequency based feature is proposed and validated to distinguish with S1 and S2 (Section 4.3.2). Another parameter can be tested by applying another windows type at the S-transform like the arbitrary and varying shape window [13]. A combination of several features can also be used to classify S1 and S2 more accurately. This can be performed by combining the α parameter with the TF_Features vector (see section 4.3.1). Then a feature selection algorithm becomes necessary to select the most accurate features.

On another hand, the classification of normal and pathological heart sounds is the final objective of any heart sounds auto-diagnosis framework. The classification rate will depend first on the segmentation results, which was the main objective of this book chapter. Then classic steps of feature extraction, feature selection, designing and testing classification systems, will be needed to complete the classification process

5.2. Real time application

One of the objectives of this study is to develop an auto diagnosis for various situations encountered in cardiology in real time. However, the S-Transform that can be considered as the heart of the proposed segmentation framework, suffers from a high computational burden. The implementation of a fast S-Transform algorithm on FPGA or GPU card will be necessary.

5.3. Sociological and psychological aspect

Introducing a smart stethoscope as a monitoring tool for home use, involves new problems related to sociological and psychological aspect of the user (patient). A smart stethoscope is a tool to facilitate the diagnosis process and to make it more objective and it will never replace the cardiologist and other advanced techniques of Cardiology. This should be taken into consideration in the deployment process in a telemedicine framework for example. The ergonomic aspect of the measuring instrument, the way to display the data and to transmit it, will be more than necessary elements to any future tool, simple for home use by the general public for the purpose of auto-diagnosis, monitoring and warning in case of necessity.

6. Conclusion

In this book chapter, a robust module for heart sounds segmentation has been proposed. The module is divided into three blocks; localization, boundaries detection, and classification of heart sounds (S1 and S2). Several methods are proposed during this study:

- A heart sounds localization method based on the S-transform and Shannon Energy, named SSE, is proposed and evaluated against white additive Gaussian noise.
- A method for boundaries detection named OSSE is proposed. It is based on an optimization process for the energy concentration in the TF domain provided by the S-transform.
- A feature extraction methods based on Singular Value Decomposition (SVD) technique to distinguish between S1 and S2 are examined. The parameters used in the time-frequency optimization process to determine the boundaries of each extracted sound are also investigated and validated as discriminative features between S1 and S2.

Dividing the proposed segmentation method into three separate blocks, enable us to perform a targeted optimization at each level. This confers the feature of robustness to the proposed module, which is a more than necessary element to any auto-diagnosis module applicable in real life conditions.

The main objective of this study is to present a robust and generic PCG segmentation method useful in real life conditions (clinical use, home care, professional use ...). The methods in the proposed framework are evaluated on a real data (80 subjects) with different noise levels and they are validated by the cardiologist.

More robustness tests against noisy signals, algorithms complexity, facility of implementation and more signals, would contribute to optimize the proposed module.

Author details

Ali Moukadem and Alain Dieterlen
MIPS Laboratory, University of Haute Alsace, Mulhouse, France

Ali Moukadem and Christian Brandt
University Hospital of Strasbourg, CIC, Inserm, Strasbourg, France

7. References

[1] Christer Ahlstrom, NonLinear Phonocardiographic Signal Processing thesis, Link¨oping University, SE-581 85 Link¨oping, Sweden, April 2008.
[2] H Liang, S Lukkarinen, I Hartimo, Heart Sound Segmentation Algorithm Based on Heart Sound Envelogram, Helsinki University of Technology, Espoo, Finland.
[3] Samjin Choi, Zhongwei Jiang, Compariason of envelope extraction algorithms for cardiac sound signal segmentation, Micro-Mechatronics Laboratory, Yamaguchi University, 2006, Japan.
[4] Schmidt, S.E., Holst-Hansen, C., Graff, C., Toft, E., Struijk, J.J.Segmentation of heart sound recordings by a duration-dependent hidden Markov model (2010) Physiological Measurement, 31 (4), pp. 513-529.
[5] A. Moukadem, A. Dieterlen, N. Hueber, C. Brandt, Comparative study of heart sounds localization, Bioelectronics, Biomedical and Bio-inspired Systems SPIE N° 8068A-27, Prague.
[6] A. Moukadem, A. Dieterlen, N. Hueber, C. Brandt, 15TH NORDIC-BALTIC CONFERENCE ON BIOMEDICAL ENGINEERING AND MEDICAL PHYSICS (NBC 2011) IFMBE Proceedings, 2011, Volume 34, 168-171, DOI: 10.1007/978-3-642-21683-1_42.
[7] Amir A. Sepheri, et al., A nouvel method for pediatric heart sound segmentation without using the ECG, Comput. Methods Programes Biomed. (2009), doi:10.1016/j.cmpb.2009.10.006
[8] Stockwell R.G., Mansinha L., Lowe R.P., Localization of the com-plex spectrum: the S-transform, IEEE Trans. Sig. Proc. 44 (4) (1996) 998–1001.
[9] H. Liang, S. Lukkarinen, I. Hartimo, "A boundary modification method for heart sound segmentation algorithm", Computers in Cardiology, pp.593-595, 13-16 Sept., 1998.
[10] Samit Ari, Prashant Kumar, and Goutam Saha, On An Algorithm for Boundary Estimation of Commonly Occurring Heart Valve Diseases in Time Domain, India Conference, 2006 Annual IEEE, 10.1109/INDCON.2006.302758

[11] Robert C. Schlant and R. wayne Alexander (editors), "The Heart Arteries and veins", 8th ed., vol. 1, McGraw Hill Inc., 1994, Ch. 11.

[12] P. D.McFadden, J. G. Cook, and L. M. Forster, "Decomposition of gear vibration signals by the generalized S-transform," Mechanical Systems and Signal Processing, vol. 13, no. 5, pp.691–707, 1999.

[13] C. R. Pinnegar and L. Mansinha, "The S-transform with windows of arbitrary and varying shape," *Geophysics*, vol. 68, no. 1, pp. 381–385, 2003.

[14] Ervin Sejdi´c, Igor Djurovi´c, and Jin Jiang, A Window Width Optimized S-Transform, EURASIP Journal on Advances in Signal Processing, Volume 2008, Article ID 672941, 13 pages doi:10.1155/2008/672941

[15] K. Gr¨ochenig, Foundations of Time-Frequency Analysis, Birkh¨auser, Boston, Mass, USA, 2001.

[16] LJ. Stankovi´c, "Measure of some time-frequency distributions concentration," *Signal Processing*, vol. 81, no. 3, pp. 621–631, 2001.

[17] Dokur Z., Ölmez T., Feature determination for heart sounds based on divergence analysis, Digital Signal Process. (2007),doi:10.1016/j.dsp. 2007.11.003.

[18] Yan Z. et al., The moment segmentation analysis of heart sound pattern, Comput. Methods Programs Biomed.(2009),doi:10.1016/j.cmppb.2009.09.008.

[19] Marinovic M. and Eichmann G., Feature extraction and pattern classification in space-spatial frequency domain. In SPIE Intelligent Robots and Computer Vision, pages 19–25, 1985.

[20] Hassanpour H., Mesbah M., Boashash B.. Time-frequency feature extraction of newborn EEG seizure using svd-based techniques. Eurasip J Appl Sig Proc, 16:2544-2554, 2004.

[21] Ahlstrom C., Hult P., Rask P., Karlsson J-E, Nylander E, Dahlstr¨om U, Ask P: Feature Extraction for Systolic Heart Murmur Classification. Annals of Biomedical Engineering. 2006. 34(11):1666-1677.

[22] He L., Lech M., Maddage C. N., Allen N., Study of empirical mode decomposition and spectral analysis for stress and emotion classification in natural speech, Biomedical signal processing an control 6 (2011) 139-146.

[23] Liang H., Lin Z., MCCallum R., Application of the Empirical Mode Decomposition to the Analysis of Esophageal Manometric Data in Gastroesophageal Relfux Disease, IEEE T. Biomedl. Eng., 52(10), 1692 – 1701, 2005.

[24] Charleston-Villalobos S., Aljama-Corrales, A. T., González-Camarena R., Analysis of Simulated Heart Sounds by Intrinsic Mode Functions, Proceedings of the 28th IEEE EMBS Annual International onferenceNew York City, USA, Aug 30-Sept 3, 2006.

[25] Liu L., Wang H., Wang Y., Tao T., Wu X., Feature Analysis of Heart Sound Based on the Improved Hilbert-Huang Transform, 3rd IEEE International Conference on Computer Science and Information Technology (ICCSIT), 2010.

[26] A. Moukadem, A. Dieterlen, N. Hueber, C. Brandt, Study of two feature extraction methods to distinguish between the first and the second heart sounds, International Conference on Bio-inspired Systems and Signal Processing, BIOSIGNALS 2012.